WEIGHT LOSS

AN 8-WEEK PLAN FOR LOSING WEIGHT AND STAYING HEALTHY

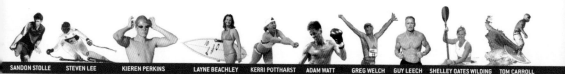

SANDON STOLLE   STEVEN LEE   KIEREN PERKINS   LAYNE BEACHLEY   KERRI POTTHARST   ADAM WATT   GREG WELCH   GUY LEECH   SHELLEY OATES WILDING   TOM CARROLL

funtastic™

First published in Australia by Funtastic Limited, 2004

1076 Centre Road, South Oakleigh
Victoria 3167, Australia

Ph: 61 3 9579 6011 Fax: 61 3 9576 4048
www.funtastic.com.au
Email: publishing@funtastic.com.au

Written by Sharon Natoli and Tony Boutagy
Contributions by Lisa Westlake
Art Direction by Rose Markovic
Designed by Rose Markovic and Ivan Finnegan
Edited by Joanne Lomasney and Gillian Hutchison
Photography by Mark Donaldson and Ned Meldrum
Hair & Make-up by Tira Jaye, Amy Corridan and Michelle Brown

Printed and bound in China
1 2 3 4 5 6 7 8 9 10

Natoli, Sharon.

Fitsmart weightloss: an 8-week plan for losing weight and
staying healthy.

1. Weight loss. 2. Health. I. Boutagy, Tony. II. Donaldson, Mark,
1959-. III. Title

ISBN 1 74111 796 8.

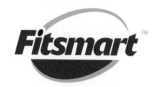

WEIGHT LOSS

AN 8-WEEK PLAN FOR LOSING WEIGHT AND STAYING HEALTHY

SHARON NATOLI AND TONY BOUTAGY

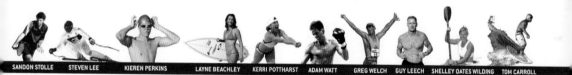

SANDON STOLLE   STEVEN LEE   KIEREN PERKINS   LAYNE BEACHLEY   KERRI POTTHARST   ADAM WATT   GREG WELCH   GUY LEECH   SHELLEY OATES WILDING   TOM CARROLL

funtastic™

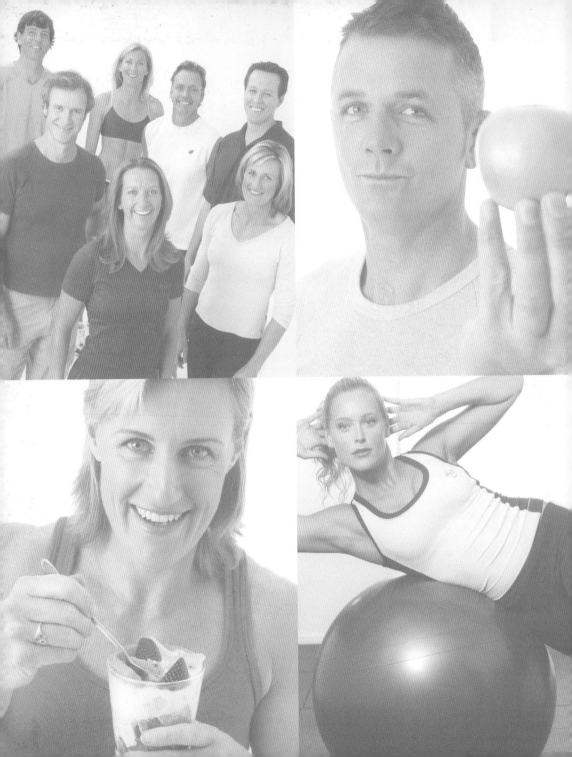

contents

introduction

Australia is a country renowned for its active, outdoor-focused culture, and one that has produced world-class champion athletes who dominate many sports. Despite this, Australia has the third highest level of obesity in the world. In fact, we have the single highest growth rate of obesity worldwide.

To combat this problem, some of Australia's leading sporting identities joined forces to establish a system of health and fitness that is fun and accessible.

The result is Fitsmart—a structured and customised fitness and nutrition program. These world champion athletes are living proof you can achieve what you set your mind to. These athletes are the backbone of Fitsmart and their collective experiences and knowledge provide a wealth of information, making Fitsmart a reliable and uniquely Australian health and fitness authority.

THE FITSMART PHILOSOPHY

The Fitsmart approach is based around the secrets of world champion athletes and leading nutritionist and fitness experts. The Fitsmart philosophy focuses on Fitness, Food, and Motivation as the core ingredients to embrace and maintain a healthy lifestyle.

To make it easy for you, we provide straightforward advice to apply to your busy lifestyle. We don't recommend unusual foods, strict regimes, or magic potions. We do recommend gradual, realistic, and practical changes you can maintain over the long term—after all, why be healthy for just 2 months when you've got the rest of your life to enjoy?

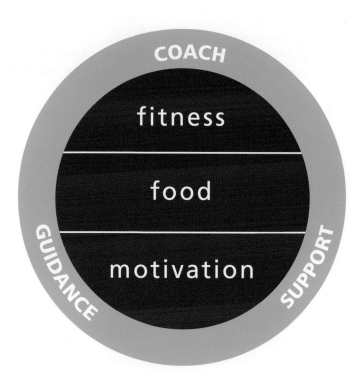

WHO IS FITSMART?

KIEREN PERKINS
Age: 29
Birthplace: Brisbane
Olympic Gold Medallist
- Swimming

ADAM WATT
Age: 34
Birthplace: Sydney
Commonwealth Boxing
Champion

GUY LEECH
Age: 38
Birthplace: Melbourne
World Ironman Champion

SANDON STOLLE
Age: 32
Birthplace: Grafton
US Open Doubles Champion

TOM CARROLL
Age: 41
Birthplace: Sydney
World Surfing Champion

SHELLEY OATES WILDING
Age: 37
Birthplace: Sydney
Dual Olympian - Kayaking

LAYNE BEACHLEY
Age: 30
Birthplace: Sydney
World Surfing Champion

STEVEN LEE
Age: 40
Birthplace: Sydney
World Cup SuperG Winner

GREG WELCH
Age: 38
Birthplace: Sydney
World Sprint Triathlon
Champion

KERRI POTTHARST
Age: 39
Birthplace: Adelaide
Olympic Gold Medallist -
Beach Volleyball

SHARON NATOLI

Bachelor of Science, Bachelor of Nutrition and Dietetics.

Sharon Natoli is an Accredited Practising Dietitian and Founding Director of Food and Nutrition Australia. Sharon commenced her career as a dietitian in 1989 and frequently presents at conferences and regularly appears on television programs and in leading magazines.

FOOD & NUTRITION AUSTRALIA

All of Fitsmart's nutrition information is independently reviewed by FNA.

For further information visit their website at **www.foodnut.com.au**

Established in 1997, Food & Nutrition Australia provies professional nutrition services for individuals, groups, the media, and the food industry.

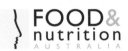

TONY BOUTAGY

Bachelor of Human Movement Studies. Undertaking post-graduate research in Exercise Science.

Tony Boutagy is a Strength and Conditioning Coach based in Sydney. In addition to writing books and numerous magazine articles, Tony lectures in Australia and internationally on all aspects of performance enhancement, strength, fitness, and weight loss. He is the winner of the 2004 Australian Fitness Industry Author of the Year award.

HOW TO USE THIS BOOK

This book is a guide to achievable and effective weight loss. The principles of Fitsmart—Food, Fitness, and Motivation—will help you reduce fat and develop healthy eating and exercise patterns for life.

There are 3 different weight loss programs to satisfy a broad range of goals:

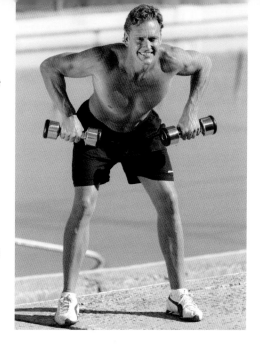

PLAN A:

MAKE A START. This program is for people who are very overweight, have poor eating habits, and are relatively new to exercising.

PLAN B:

GET IN SHAPE. This program is for those people who want to lose some excess weight and become more energised through an improved diet and strengthening exercises.

PLAN C:

FIRM UP FOR LIFE. This program is targeted at people who are already active but want to tone up and look trim.

The food programs allow for flexibility and freedom, and encourage you to have total control over your diet. You will be more likely to stick to an eating plan you create, than one where you are told to eat a certain food on a certain day.

The exercise programs are simple and easy to use, and are broken down into 2-week blocks. The strength exercises only change every 2 weeks and the cardiovascular workout times increase gradually.

These 8-week programs are realistic and safe ways to achieve weight loss. The positive effects you experience will give you all the incentive you need to make these healthier habits a way of life.

Before embarking on your weight loss program, read the whole book to decide exactly what you want. You are about to make a wonderful lifestyle change and you've taken the first step already just by opening this book.

Ask yourself honestly, 'What do I want to achieve?'

This is your long-term goal. To make the journey easier, you also need short-term goals. These may be monthly, weekly, or even daily goals, and will keep changing as you achieve them.

In the back of the book is a Contract of Commitment. Write down your goals, sign it, and keep it in a place you will see every day, like on the fridge door.

You will also find a diary page in the back. Make copies of this so you will have enough for your entire program. You can print these pages from the website: www.fitsmart. com.au. Use this diary to record everything—food, exercise, and your weekly goals. This is the best way to stay focused and is a great way to track your progress.

But most of all, enjoy the experience. Enjoy the new meals you will be eating, enjoy the new exercises, and enjoy feeling healthy.

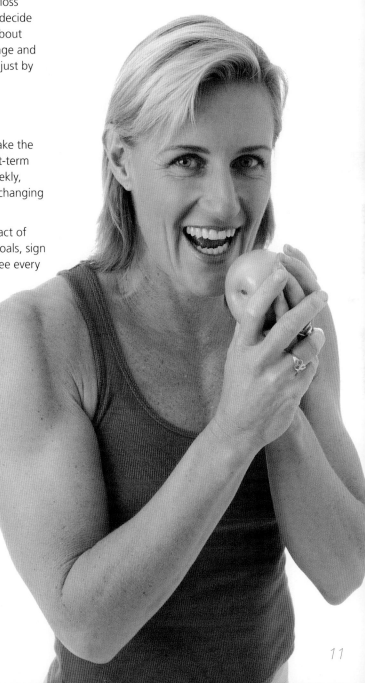

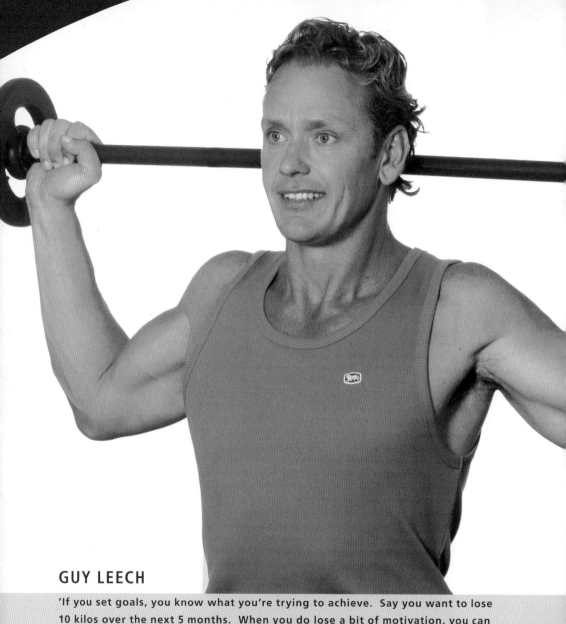

GUY LEECH

'If you set goals, you know what you're trying to achieve. Say you want to lose 10 kilos over the next 5 months. When you do lose a bit of motivation, you can go back and think about why you're doing it in the first place.'

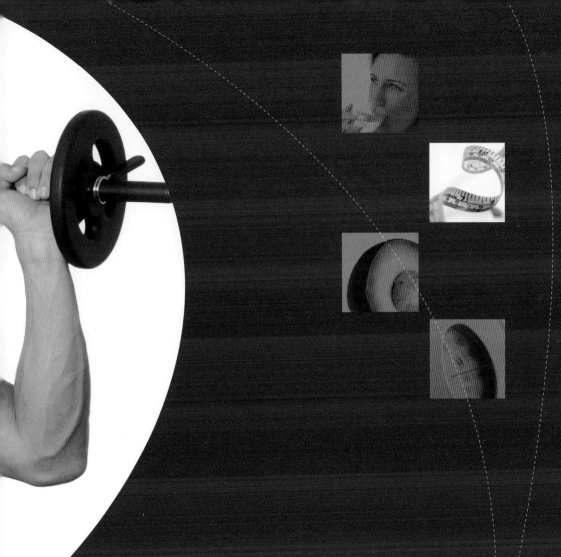

WEIGHT &
WEIGHT LOSS

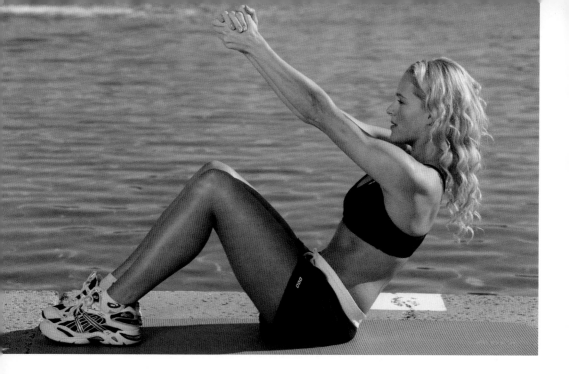

Despite decades of research, we still don't fully understand why some people gain weight more easily than others. Genetics appear to play an important role, but it is likely the most important factor is the environment. To lose weight, you must ensure the level of physical activity burns up more energy than what you take in. The importance of physical activity cannot be over-emphasised, not only in weight control, but for general health and fitness.

Controlling the amount of energy (measured in kilojoules) in the diet is vital to weight loss. This involves awareness of fat content of foods, reading food labels, and limiting portion sizes of high-fat and kilojoule-laden foods.

For weight loss to be maintained, you should aim to lose weight slowly and steadily—about 1kg per fortnight.

WEIGHT REDUCTION STEPS

- **Manage portion sizes and total kilojoule intake.**
- **Reduce fatty and sugary foods.**
- **Monitor alcohol intake.**
- **Increase physical activity.**
- **Commence a program of structured physical activity that gradually increases both volume and intensity of exercise.**

The most important goal is to achieve a weight and body shape healthy for you.

BODY WEIGHT

Your weight on the scales is one way of assessing whether you are within a healthy weight range. Body mass index (BMI) is used to estimate the best weight range for your health. It is calculated by dividing your weight in kilograms by your height in metres squared.

In many cases, your BMI relates closely to body fat. However, sometimes you also need to measure your percentage body fat and/or waist measurement to obtain an accurate picture. This is particularly true if you are already close to, or within, your healthy weight range.

SOME EXCEPTIONS

BMI does not differentiate between body fat and muscle mass. For example, muscly people may have a high BMI, but are not overweight, and people who can't move around a lot may have muscle wasting and high percentage body fat, but a low BMI.

For people of Asian origins, who have a relatively lower average height, the cut-offs for being overweight and obese are lower. For these people, there is an increased risk of diabetes and cardiovascular disease with a BMI as low as 23. In taller Caucasian populations, this risk occurs around a BMI of 27.

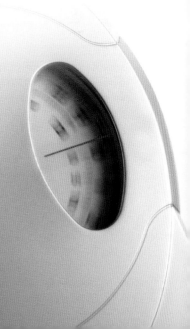

BODY MASS INDEX

HEIGHT	19	20	21	22	23	24	25	26	27	28	29	30	35	40
						WEIGHT (KILOGRAMS)								
1.47m (4'10")	41	43	45	47	50	52	54	56	59	61	63	65	76	87
1.50m (4'11")	43	45	47	49	52	54	56	58	60	63	65	67	78	89
1.52m (5'0")	44	46	49	51	54	55	58	60	63	65	67	69	81	93
1.55m (5'1")	45	48	50	53	55	58	60	62	65	67	69	72	84	96
1.57m (5'2")	47	49	52	54	57	59	62	64	67	69	72	74	87	99
1.60m (5'3")	49	51	54	56	59	61	64	66	69	71	74	77	89	102
1.63m (5'4")	50	53	55	58	61	64	66	68	71	74	77	79	93	105
1.65m (5'5")	52	54	57	60	63	65	68	71	74	76	79	82	95	109
1.68m (5'6")	54	56	59	62	64	67	70	73	76	78	81	84	98	112
1.70m (5'7")	55	58	61	64	66	69	72	75	78	81	84	87	101	116
1.73m (5'8")	57	59	63	65	68	72	74	78	80	83	86	89	104	119
1.75m (5'9")	58	61	64	68	70	73	77	80	83	86	89	92	107	122
1.78m (5'10")	60	63	66	69	72	76	79	82	85	88	92	94	110	126
1.80m (5'11")	62	65	68	71	75	78	81	84	88	90	94	98	113	130
1.83m (6'0")	64	67	70	74	77	80	83	87	90	93	97	100	117	133
1.85m (6'1")	65	68	72	75	79	83	86	89	93	96	99	103	120	137
1.88m (6'2")	67	70	74	78	81	84	88	92	95	99	102	106	123	141
1.90m (6'3")	69	73	76	80	83	87	91	94	98	102	105	108	127	145
1.93m (6'4")	71	74	78	82	86	89	93	97	100	104	108	112	130	149

Rating

Underweight:	Less than 18.5
Normal weight:	18.5 – 24.9
Overweight:	25 – 29.9
Obese:	30 or more

Remember, BMI is only an approximate measure of the best weight for health.

SETTING A GOAL WEIGHT

While weight for height charts can be useful, they may not always be appropriate for you. Set a goal weight using any of the following methods.

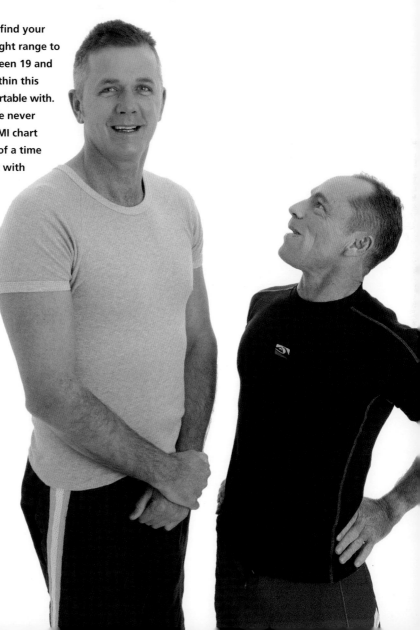

- **Using the BMI chart, find your height. Find the weight range to give you a BMI between 19 and 25. Pick a weight within this range you feel comfortable with.**
- **If you know you have never weighed what the BMI chart is telling you, think of a time when you felt happy with your weight and set this as your goal.**
- **Research shows if you lose 10% of your body weight, you experience significant improvements in your health. Losing 10% of your weight is a great goal to begin with.**

Most importantly, be realistic with your goal weight and remember changing your weight won't change your genetically predetermined body shape.

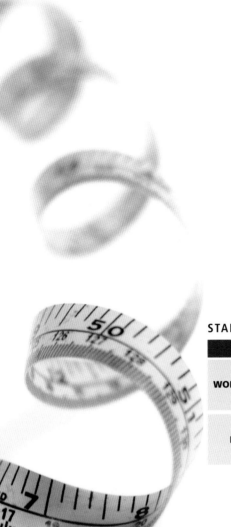

BODY FAT

When we talk about weight loss, we're really talking about fat loss. Losing weight as a result of burning up fat stores is the key aim. Excess body fat lies beneath the skin and around internal organs and it is this body fat that is associated with many people's dissatisfaction with how they look and feel. To monitor body fat loss, you need to measure the percentage of body fat you carry. To do this, you need scales that perform this measure, or a trained health or fitness professional to perform the pinch test using skin fold callipers. Ask at your local gym.

The table below provides a guide to ideal percentage body fat measures for different ages:

STANDARD BODY FAT RANGES FOR ADULTS

	AGE	UNDERFAT	HEALTHY	OVERFAT	OBESE
WOMEN	20-39	21-33%	21-33%	33-39%	38%+
	40-59	23-34%	23-34%	34-40%	40%+
	60-79	24-36%	24-36%	36-42%	42%+
MEN	20-39	8-20%	8-20%	20-25%	25%+
	40-59	11-22%	11-22%	22-28%	28%+
	60-79	13-25%	13-25%	25-30%	30%+

Setting yourself a goal for reducing percentage body fat if you are 'overfat' is highly recommended. This is even more important than focusing on total body weight. You can reduce your percentage of body fat by either increasing muscle, or losing fat. A combination of both is the ideal approach and can be achieved through the Fitsmart Weight Loss programs.

BODY FAT DISTRIBUTION

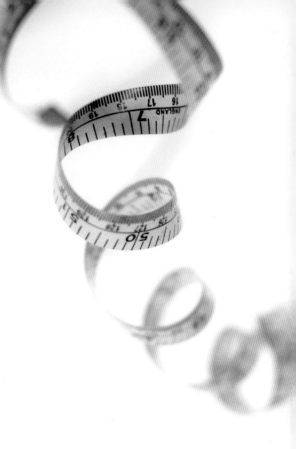

When it comes to health, it is not only the amount of weight and body fat you carry that's important, but where you carry it. Body fat distributed around the stomach is associated with an increased risk of diabetes, high blood pressure, high cholesterol, and cardiovascular disease. Fat deposited around the hips and buttocks doesn't have this same risk. For this reason, measuring your waist circumference is an important measure.

Men – Place the tape measure around your middle, over your belly button. Make sure your belly button points forward.

Women – Measure the smallest part of your waist between the top of your hip bones and the last rib.

Waist Measure (cm)		
RISK LEVEL	MEN	WOMEN
Increased risk	94	94
Substantially increased risk	102	102

Generally, the association between health risks and body fat distribution is as follows:

- **Least risk - slim with no pot belly.**
- **Moderate risk - overweight with no pot belly.**
- **Moderate-high risk - slim with pot belly.**
- **High risk - overweight with pot belly.**

Where fat is distributed in the body is influenced by your genetic make-up. However, keeping physically active, avoiding smoking, and choosing unsaturated rather than saturated fat have all been shown to decrease the risk of developing a fat tummy.

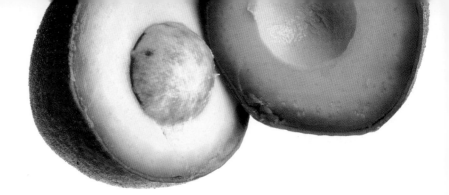

A healthy and balanced diet plays a major role in the prevention of many lifestyle-related diseases.

▶ *Heart disease*

Being overweight can cause high levels of a type of fat found in the bloodstream called triglycerides which increases the risk of heart disease. Being overweight also increases the 'bad' LDL cholesterol and raises blood pressure. Weight reduction and following a diet low in saturated fat can significantly lower cholesterol and triglyceride levels and lowers blood pressure.

▶ *Diabetes*

Having adult-onset, or Type 2 diabetes, greatly increases the risk of heart disease. Weight management is vital to blood glucose control and improves the body's ability to use insulin, which is needed to gain energy from carbohydrates.

▶ *Cancer*

A healthy diet combined with regular physical activity can reduce cancer rates by up to a third. Being overweight increases your risk of developing kidney, endometrial, bowel, and breast cancers.

▶ *Arthritis*

Obesity is a risk factor for osteoarthritis, the most common form of arthritis. Along with weight reduction, Omega-3 fats found in fish can be useful in easing symptoms of rheumatoid arthritis.

▶ *PCOS (Polycystic Ovarian Syndrome)*

The benefits of weight management for women with PCOS include improved fertility, improved insulin sensitivity and blood glucose control, and improved blood pressure levels.

▶ *Blood pressure*

Being overweight increases your risk of developing high blood pressure by 2-6 times. Weight loss can reduce the need for medication to control blood pressure. A high intake of salt (sodium) and a low intake of potassium (found largely in fruits and vegetables) are also associated with increased blood pressure levels.

WEIGHT LOSS

Weight loss can occur when the body loses fat, fluid, carbohydrate stores, or muscle. Ideally, when you lose weight most of it will be from fat stores. Fat loss occurs when the body needs to draw on its energy reserves to provide fuel for daily activities, including exercise. To achieve this, you need to eat fewer kilojoules than your body burns up in a day. By eating less and exercising more you will begin to burn fat. However, fat burning is a gradual process. Slow and steady is the ideal approach for effective weight loss.

Certain fad diets promote rapid loss of weight. Any sudden weight loss is usually due to the body losing fluid as a result of rapid breakdown of carbohydrate stores. Each gram of carbohydrate stored in the body is stored with 2.7g of water. On a low-carbohydrate diet, the weight on the scales will drop quickly in the first few weeks—due to the breakdown of carbohydrates and subsequent loss of stored fluid. This 'weight loss' quickly becomes 'weight gain' when you return to normal eating habits.

The ideal rate of weight loss is 0.5-1kg a week. This rate is more likely to result in a reduction of body fat and is also more likely to result in the weight staying off for the long-term. If you are losing 0.5kg of body fat per week, you can expect a reduction in body fat of around 2% a month. This will be higher if you gain muscle at the same time.

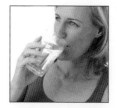

MAINTAINING WEIGHT LOSS

Long-term weight loss means making changes you can maintain for life. It is not feasible to stay on a 'diet' for life, so consider your weight loss eating pattern as a healthy approach to eating you will adopt over time. It is more important to lose a few kilos and maintain the weight loss over a lifetime, than to lose weight quickly only to regain it.

Successful weight loss tips

‣ **Follow a personal eating plan**
‣ **Exercise regularly**
‣ **Monitor your weight regularly**
‣ **Monitor your food intake**
‣ **Eat breakfast**
‣ **Eat a low-fat diet**
‣ **Manage stress effectively**

Women, in particular, will be more successful in maintaining their weight loss if they undertake long, regular (although not necessarily vigorous) exercise, such as walking.

Adopting habits that will benefit in the long term is very important. The meal plans and recipes in this book are a guide to getting you on the right track. If you find you can only make some changes, that's fine. Aim to achieve 80% of what is recommended and you'll be well on the way to a new, fitter, and healthier you.

FAT INTAKE

Fat provides the highest amount of energy (kilojoules) per gram compared with protein, carbohydrate, and alcohol. To lose weight, it is therefore important to consider how much fat you eat.

Fatty foods don't fill you up as quickly as carbohydrate and protein-rich foods. This means it's easier to overeat high-fat foods and this can be a major reason why many people gain weight over time.

The introduction of low-fat foods in supermarkets makes it easier to maintain a diet low in fat. However, beware of low-fat processed foods as the fat is often replaced by sugars. These low-fat foods may be lower in kilojoules than their usual counterparts but are often low in nutrients as well. Instead, consider enjoying the usual higher fat varieties in moderation and be sure to read labels and compare products when selecting foods.

HIGH-FAT FOODS

Donuts, cakes, pastries, biscuits, chocolate, deep-fried foods, cheese, pizza, sausages, salami, devon, butter, cream, creamy salad dressings.

LOW-FAT, HIGH-SUGAR FOODS

Biscuits, cakes, muffins, ice-cream, confectionery, slices, 'health' bars.

Minimise both these types of foods in your daily eating plan.

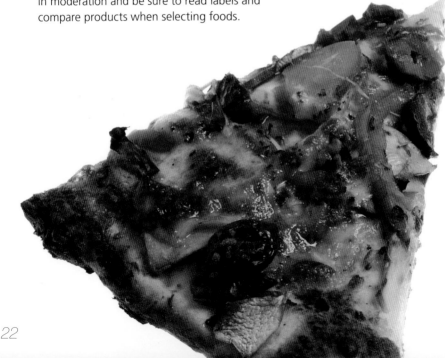

HOW MUCH FAT?

The National Health and Medical Research Council recommends an eating pattern where around 30% of our kilojoules come from fat. This equates to approximately 40-65g of fat per day for women and 55-85g of fat per day for men.

A small amount of fat is vital for good health. Healthy fats supply essential fatty acids and are carriers for fat-soluble vitamins and antioxidants. However, eating too much fat will make it harder to lose weight. Eating too much saturated fat can contribute to lifestyle-related diseases such as high blood cholesterol and Type 2 diabetes. Make sure the fats you do include in your diet are mostly polyunsaturated or monounsaturated types, e.g., olive oil, nuts, avocado, and seeds.

WAYS TO BALANCE FAT INTAKE

- Minimise saturated fats. This includes full-cream milk, yoghurt, cheese, butter, cream, sour cream, coconut milk, coconut cream, fat on meat, bacon, and chicken skin.
- Use low-fat dairy products. Try skim or reduced-fat varieties.
- Beware of 'hidden' saturated fats. Minimise your intake of chips, biscuits, fast foods, fried takeaways, processed meats, pies, pastries, quiches, creamy sauces, and chocolate.
- Use fat-reduced or light margarine.
- Use healthy oils in moderation. These include olive, peanut, canola, soy bean, safflower, corn, sunflower, grapeseed, cottonseed, and sesame. Heat the pan before adding oil, or try an oil spray.
- Instead of butter, spread bread with a little olive oil, avocado, peanut butter, or polyunsaturated or monounsaturated margarine.
- Eat a small handful of unsalted nuts as a snack.
- Eat at least 2 fish meals a week.
- Use low-fat cooking methods such as grilling, microwaving, steaming, barbecuing, stir-frying, or baking.
- Season food with garlic, ginger, chilli, chutney, balsamic vinegar, lemon juice, mustard, Worcestershire, soy or teriyaki sauces, herbs and spices, pepper or seasoning mixtures.
- For roasting vegetables, steam or microwave first, then spray or brush with a little healthy oil and bake. Alternatively, roast vegetables on a tray lined with baking paper.
- Chill casseroles, curries, and soups. Skim fat from the surface before reheating.
- Choose restaurant foods low in fat. Look for seafood, grilled meats, stir-fries, tomato or vegetable sauces, salads, soups, or lean meat and salad sandwiches.

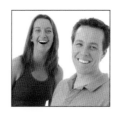

DETERMINING KILOJOULE REQUIREMENTS

Once you start your program and monitor your progress, the rate of weight loss will provide a good indication of whether you are at the right kilojoule level. As a starting point, see the table below to work out your daily kilojoule requirements.

The tables are based on a lifestyle of low physical activity such as office work and 30 minutes exercise once or twice a week.

For weight loss, subtract 2100kJ from your daily requirement. For example:

FEMALE

Current weight 75kg

Age 35 years

For weight maintenance 7560kJ per day

For weight loss 7560kJ-2100kJ = 5460kJ per day

NOTE FOR THOSE WHO ARE ACTIVE

Active people will need to eat more kilojoules than outlined below. If you undertake an hour of moderate to high intensity exercise around 5 times a week, or have a very active job, add 1500 kilojoules to your daily total as calculated above.

Females – daily kilojoule requirements to maintain weight

CURRENT WEIGHT	Age			
	20-30	30-40	40-50	50-60
65-80kg	7560kJ	7560kJ	7390kJ	7140kJ
80-100kg	8570kJ	8400kJ	7980kJ	7850kJ
100-120kg	9240kJ	9240kJ	8820kJ	8820kJ
>120kg	10080kJ	9660kJ	9580kJ	9320kJ

Males – daily kilojoule requirements to maintain weight

CURRENT WEIGHT	Age			
	20-30	30-40	40-50	50-60
65-80kg	8650kJ	8360kJ	7980kJ	7850kJ
80-100kg	9200kJ	8900kJ	8900kJ	8360kJ
100-120kg	10080kJ	10080kJ	9660KJ	9660kJ
>120kg	10500kJ	10500kJ	10080kJ	10080kJ

DIFFERENT APPROACHES TO WEIGHT LOSS

The Fitsmart plans are designed around various levels of activity and degrees of weight loss. They are also designed to give the option of following a higher protein, low-fat eating plan, or a higher carbohydrate, low-fat eating plan. The plan for you depends on where you are now and your weight goal. Use the following questionnaire to choose the most appropriate plan for you.

1. **HOW WOULD YOU RATE YOUR CURRENT LEVEL OF ACTIVITY?**
    a) Sedentary (no planned exercise)
    b) Moderately active (moderate level exercise 2-3 times a week)
    c) Quite active (moderate to high level exercise 4 or more times a week)

2. **HOW MUCH WEIGHT DO YOU WANT TO LOSE?**
    a) More than 20kg
    b) 10-20kg
    c) Less than 10kg

3. **TO LOSE WEIGHT, YOU THINK YOU NEED TO:**
    a) Change your eating habits quite significantly
    b) Keep eating the same foods but eat a bit less than usual
    c) Cut down on the extras to see results (chocolate, alcohol, lollies, etc)

4. **THE KEY MOTIVATING FORCE FOR YOU TO LOSE WEIGHT IS:**
    a) To see my toes when I look down
    b) To feel energised
    c) To tone up and look trim

5. **I USUALLY LOSE WEIGHT WHEN I:**
    a) Cut out the junk foods I eat
    b) Cut down on my portion sizes and increase my activity level
    c) Cut out the extras that creep in too often

RESULTS:

If you answered mostly a, the best plan for you is Fitsmart Plan A.

If you answered mostly b, the best plan for you is Fitsmart Plan B.

If you answered mostly C, the best plan for you is Fitsmart Plan C.

Plan B and Plan C have the option of a higher protein or a higher carbohydrate eating pattern. Have a look at the meal plans and decide which style of eating you will most likely stick to. You can switch between a higher carbohydrate eating plan and a higher protein eating plan for variety. However, you must follow one plan for an entire day to ensure adequate nutrition.

People with any of the following are likely to benefit from a higher protein eating plan:

▸ **High levels of triglycerides in the blood.**
▸ **Most of their body fat deposited around their middle.**
▸ **Elevated blood glucose levels or Type 2 diabetes.**
▸ **Low levels of the type of cholesterol called HDL cholesterol.**

IMPORTANT NOTE: Check with your general practitioner before starting on a Fitsmart program if you have a medical condition.

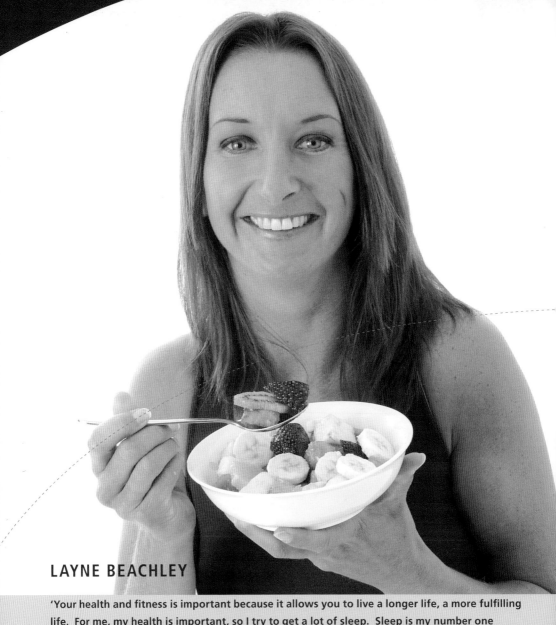

LAYNE BEACHLEY

'Your health and fitness is important because it allows you to live a longer life, a more fulfilling life. For me, my health is important, so I try to get a lot of sleep. Sleep is my number one priority. A good diet is my second priority.'

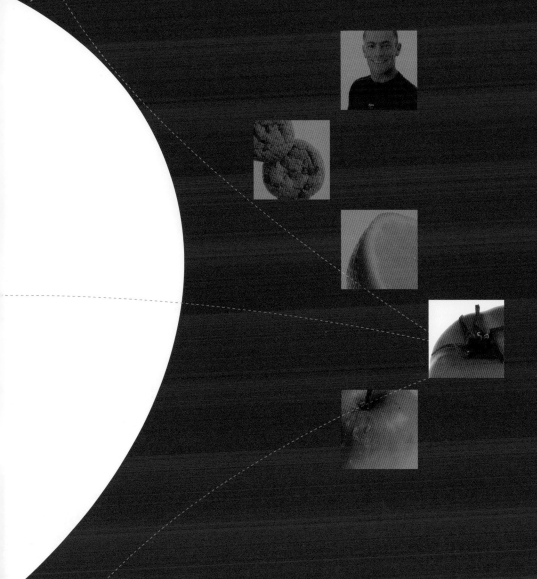

FOOD

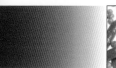

weight loss and eating habits

EATING BREAKFAST

Breakfast is the most important meal of the day. It refuels your body, gets your metabolism working, and improves energy levels throughout the morning.

Research shows people who eat breakfast find it easier to control their weight. Eating breakfast also helps manage hunger. Just skipping breakfast can result in a 2.5kg weight increase in a year. By starting your day with breakfast, you'll find it easier to follow a healthy eating plan for weight loss.

The Fitsmart meal plans provide a range of delicious options for breakfast. If lack of time is the reason you skip breakfast, set your alarm 15 minutes earlier. It also helps to avoid overeating at night so you wake with a good appetite. Exercising before breakfast can also increase your appetite in the morning.

EATING REGULARLY

Eating regularly throughout the day helps control appetite and prevents overeating at meal times, so plan to eat something healthy every 3-5 hours. It's important to plan meals and snacks to enable you to do this.

VEGETABLES AND FRUIT

Vegetables are a great source of vitamins, minerals, dietary fibre, and are low in kilojoules. Bulking up your meals with extra vegetables and salad is a good way to satisfy your appetite while losing weight. Try to eat a variety of vegetables and aim to eat at least 5 handfuls a day.

Ways to enjoy vegetables

- **Vegetable soup**
- **Corn on the cob**
- **Mixed salads**
- **Grilled or baked vegetables**
- **Stir-fried vegetables**

Fruit is also a source of vitamins, minerals, and is low in fat and kilojoules. It is also high in fibre, making it a great snack. All fruit is good for you, so eat a variety and aim for at least 2 pieces daily.

Ways to enjoy fruit

- **Chop a banana on your cereal**
- **Eat fruit salad and yoghurt for a snack**
- **Crunch an apple on the run**
- **Treat yourself with a sweet, tropical fruit**
- **Poach pears for dessert**

EXCESS SUGAR

To lose weight, minimising added sugar in the diet is essential. No more than 10% of your kilojoule intake should be from added sugars. This means around 7 teaspoons a day when you are aiming to lose weight.

Added sugars include any sugar you add in tea, coffee, cooking, and baking. It also includes sugar in products you buy. The table below shows how many teaspoons of added sugar are in some common foods.

FOOD	SUGAR (TSP)
2 choc chip biscuits	1
1 donut	1.5
1 bowl sugar-sweetened breakfast cereal	2.5
1 muffin	3
2 chocolate biscuits	3.5
1 chocolate ice-cream on a stick	5
1 300ml flavoured milk	7
1 60g chocolate bar	8.5
1 can soft drink	10

SALT

While reducing salt intake will not help you lose weight, it is recommended salt be limited in the diet for good health. Too much salt has been linked with high blood pressure, fluid retention, the risk of osteoporosis, kidney problems, and premenstrual tension.

Aim to limit your daily intake to below 2000mg sodium—1 teaspoon of salt—from all sources, not just salt added to foods. Choose low-salt foods and minimise added salt in cooking.

OMEGA-3 AND FISH

Cutting out all sources of fat from the diet while trying to lose weight is unhealthy and not recommended. Omega-3 fatty acids are a type of essential polyunsaturated fat that have heart health benefits and anti-inflammatory properties. Fish is the best source of Omega-3 fats and should be included regularly in a healthy eating plan. Fish is also low in kilojoules and rich in other essential nutrients. Try to enjoy 2 fish meals a week to help meet Omega-3 fatty acids, zinc, and protein requirements.

DRINKING FLUIDS

When trying to lose weight, choosing what to drink is also important. Soft drinks and some fruit juices are high in sugar and can significantly add to your daily kilojoule intake. The best alternative is water, but if you need something sweet, choose diet cordial or diet soft drinks.

ADEQUATE FIBRE

Fibre-rich meals are digested slowly, satisfying hunger for longer. Higher fibre diets tend to reduce fat stored around the stomach.

High-fibre foods include: wholegrain breads and cereals, dried beans and peas, vegetables, fruits, dried fruit, and nuts. When losing weight, it is important to select high-fibre foods to help meet daily fibre requirements.

ALCOHOL

Alcohol is high in kilojoules so it's best to limit your intake while losing weight.

Ways to enjoy alcohol

▸ Drink light beer instead of regular strength.
▸ Mix half wine with half soda water.
▸ Mix spirits with diet soft drinks.
▸ Have a glass of water or diet soft drink between alcoholic drinks.

TAKEAWAY FOOD

Eating takeaway food makes it difficult to control fat and kilojoule intake. If eating takeaways, it's important to make healthy choices and avoid large servings.

Healthy takeaway options

▸ Sushi and sashimi.
▸ Clear soups with vegetables, noodles, seafood, tofu, lean meat or chicken.
▸ Stir-fries with lean meat, chicken, seafood or tofu, and plenty of vegetables.
▸ Meat dishes grilled, barbecued, or braised.
▸ Steamed or boiled rice.
▸ Grilled fish with salad.
▸ Sandwiches or wraps with wholemeal or wholegrain bread. Choose fillings such as lean meats, tuna, salmon, cottage or ricotta cheese, and salad or grilled vegetables.
▸ Baked potato with chilli con carne, tuna and sweet corn, cottage cheese with mushrooms and herbs, or a tomato based sauce with spinach and olives.
▸ Salads with light dressings.

▸ Pasta and risotto dishes with a tomato-based sauce and vegetables.
▸ Soft tortillas and burritos with salsa and plenty of salad.

SPECIAL OCCASIONS

Parties and business lunches can mean three-course meals with plenty of alcohol. Making the right choices, and stopping eating when full can help keep you on track.

▸ Avoid arriving at the event overly hungry.
▸ Eat slowly and stop once you feel full.
▸ Try ordering two courses only—entrée and main; entrée and light dessert; main and light dessert; or two entrées.
▸ Choose plain or wholegrain fresh bread and side salads or vegetables with your meal.
▸ At buffets, fill your plate once for each course.
▸ Sharing dishes can increase variety and help reduce the amount eaten. Enjoy alcohol in moderation. Too many drinks can result in overeating.

PICNICS

The buffet style of picnics can be difficult to control how much you eat.

▸ Avoid pre-meal nibbles or take your own low-fat options such as pretzels, or vegetable sticks with a low-fat dip. Fill your plate once.
▸ Take fresh fruit for dessert and avoid the slices and cakes (or have half a piece).
▸ Stick to water or diet soft drinks.

PORTION CONTROL

Upgraded meal sizes and all-you-can-eat offers entice you to eat and drink more. It only takes an extra 850 kilojoules per week to add an extra 1.5kg of body fat over a year. This is the equivalent of an extra slice of cake per week.

When it comes to managing weight, being conscious of the portion size of the food you choose is as important as reading the labels for fat content.

KILOJOULE EQUIVALENT PORTIONS

BREADS AND CEREALS (600KJ)	
Wholegrain bread	1 average slice
Bagel	½ average
Fruit loaf	1 thick slice
Crumpet	1 slice
Cracker biscuits	4
Rice cakes	2½
Rice crackers	20
Cooked porridge	⅔ cup
Breakfast cereal bar	1 small
Boiled rice	½ cup
Fried rice	⅓ cup
Cooked instant noodles	½ cup
Cooked pasta	1 cup
Baked beans	½ cup

FRUIT & VEGETABLES (600KJ)	
Apple	2 small
Bananas	2 small
Grapes	2 cups
Kiwi fruit	4 small
Orange	2 medium
Mango	1 medium
Pear	2 small
Strawberries	5 cups
Watermelon	6 wedges
Rockmelon	1 medium
Fruit juice	300mL glass
Canned peaches	2 cups
Dried apricots	8
Prunes	8
Sultanas	2 tablespoons
Dried apple	8 rings
Boiled potato	1 medium
Mashed potato	⅔ cup
Steamed non-starchy green and orange vegetables	3½ cups
Sweet potato	2 x 2cm wedges
Sweet corn	1 small cob
Creamed corn	½ cup

FAST FOODS (600KJ)	
Pizza	1 small slice
Meat pie	¼ individual
Sausage roll	1½ party-sized rolls
Spring rolls	2 mini
Hamburger (junior size)	½ average
Chicken nuggets	3 pieces
Hash brown	1
Potato wedges	3 small
Hot potato chips	7 chips

MEAT AND PROTEIN FOODS (600KJ)	
Chicken breast, cooked	½ single breast
Beef steak	90g portion
Frankfurt	⅔ regular size
Ham	5 thin slices
Devon	2½ thin slices
Lamb chop	1 small chop
Hamburger rissole	1 small rissole
Grilled sausage	1 thin sausage
Crumbed fish	1 small fillet
Fish fingers	2½
Sardines	7 small
Tuna in brine	¾ cup

DAIRY (600KJ)	
Full cream milk	200mL glass
Reduced-fat milk	285mL glass
Cheddar cheese	1 slice
Cottage cheese	½ cup
Cream cheese	2 tablespoons
Reduced-fat yoghurt	150g tub
Ice-cream	2 small scoops

NUTS & SWEETS (600KJ)	
Chocolate	6 small squares
Assorted sweets	10 jubes
Almonds	20
Mixed nut	2 tablespoons
Peanut butter	1 tablespoon
Pine nuts	2 tablespoons

GLYCEMIC INDEX AND WEIGHT LOSS

The Glycemic Index (GI) is a ranking of carbohydrate containing foods based on their effect on blood glucose (blood sugar) levels. Carbohydrates that break down quickly during digestion have the highest GI values. Carbohydrates that breakdown slowly, releasing glucose gradually into the blood stream, have low GI values.

The GI is based on a ranking out of 100—low GI foods are below 55, moderate GI foods are between 55 and 70, and high GI foods are above 70.

Foods with a low GI are generally more filling and help control hunger and appetite. Many low GI foods are also high in fibre and low in fat so they satisfy your hunger by providing bulk without too many kilojoules. Low GI foods can also result in less insulin being released into the bloodstream, making it easier to lose weight. Low GI foods also provide longer lasting energy because of the slow release of glucose during digestion.

HOW TO SWITCH TO A LOW GI DIET

Try to include 1 low GI food at each meal. For example:

▸ **Use breakfast cereals based on oats, barley, and bran.**
▸ **Use wholegrain breads.**
▸ **Substitute sweet potato or corn for white potatoes.**
▸ **Eat pasta and legumes, e.g., lentils, chickpeas, and baked beans.**
▸ **Switch to basmati or doongara rice.**
▸ **Choose low GI fruits as a snack.**

There is no need to eat only low GI foods. When you eat a combination of low and high GI foods, the final GI of the meal is moderate. For example, when having baked beans (low GI) on white toast (high GI) the baked beans will lower the overall GI of the meal to a moderate level.

GLYCEMIC INDEX TABLE

FOOD	GI RATING	FOOD	GI RATING
Breads and Cereals		**Fruit**	
White bread	70	Apple	38
Wholemeal bread	77	Banana	52
Multigrain bread (9 Grain)	43	Grapes	46
Soy-Linseed bread	36	Orange	42
Corn Flakes	77	Watermelon	72
Porridge, traditional oats	51	Peach	42
Rice Bubbles®	87	Mango	51
Weet-Bix®	69	Apple juice	40
All-Bran®	30	Orange juice	53
Special K®	54	**Soups**	
Jasmine rice	109	Tomato soup	38
Basmati rice	58	Minestrone	39
Brown rice	76	Lentil soup	44
Calrose rice	83	Split pea soup	60
Pasta and Noodles		**Sugars**	
Spaghetti	38	Glucose	100
Ravioli	39	Maltose	105
Fettucine	32	Fructose	19
Instant noodles	48	Honey	44
Rice noodles	61	**Snacks**	
Gnocchi	68	Muesli bar	61
Dairy and Dairy Alternatives		Fruit roll-ups	90
Milk (full fat)	31	Pop-Tarts®	70
Skim milk	32	Popcorn	72
Chocolate milk, low-fat	34	Apricot fruit bar	50
Fruit yoghurt, low-fat	33	**Biscuits and Crackers**	
Soy milk	44	Arrowroot biscuits	69
Vanilla ice-cream, low-fat	47	Shredded wheatmeal	62
Starchy Vegetables and Legumes		Oatmeal biscuits	55
Potato	78	Snack Right Fruit Slice®	48
Mashed potato	91	Rice cakes	82
Sweet potato	44	Water cracker	78
Sweet corn	48	Ryvita®	64
Baked beans	48	Vita-Weat	55
Chickpeas	25	Crispbread	81
Lentils	29		

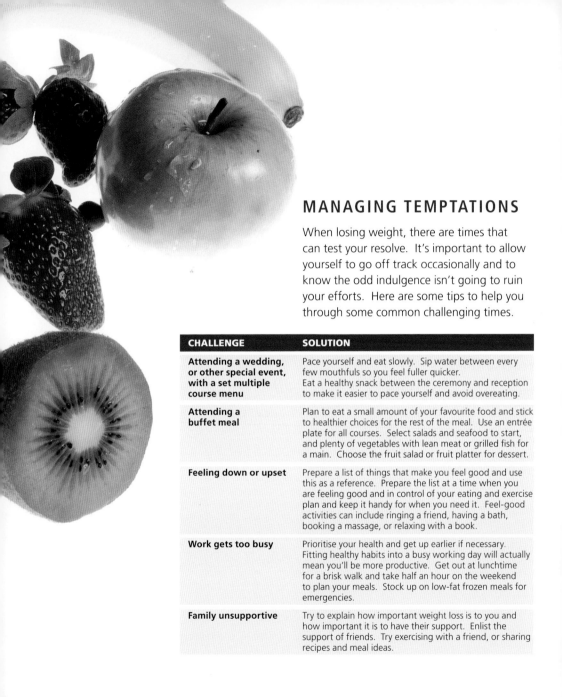

MANAGING TEMPTATIONS

When losing weight, there are times that can test your resolve. It's important to allow yourself to go off track occasionally and to know the odd indulgence isn't going to ruin your efforts. Here are some tips to help you through some common challenging times.

CHALLENGE	SOLUTION
Attending a wedding, or other special event, with a set multiple course menu	Pace yourself and eat slowly. Sip water between every few mouthfuls so you feel fuller quicker. Eat a healthy snack between the ceremony and reception to make it easier to pace yourself and avoid overeating.
Attending a buffet meal	Plan to eat a small amount of your favourite food and stick to healthier choices for the rest of the meal. Use an entrée plate for all courses. Select salads and seafood to start, and plenty of vegetables with lean meat or grilled fish for a main. Choose the fruit salad or fruit platter for dessert.
Feeling down or upset	Prepare a list of things that make you feel good and use this as a reference. Prepare the list at a time when you are feeling good and in control of your eating and exercise plan and keep it handy for when you need it. Feel-good activities can include ringing a friend, having a bath, booking a massage, or relaxing with a book.
Work gets too busy	Prioritise your health and get up earlier if necessary. Fitting healthy habits into a busy working day will actually mean you'll be more productive. Get out at lunchtime for a brisk walk and take half an hour on the weekend to plan your meals. Stock up on low-fat frozen meals for emergencies.
Family unsupportive	Try to explain how important weight loss is to you and how important it is to have their support. Enlist the support of friends. Try exercising with a friend, or sharing recipes and meal ideas.

REALISTIC EXPECTATIONS

When losing weight it is extremely important to have realistic expectations. Slow and steady is the key to long-term weight loss success, and being aware that it is normal to experience flat spots along the way can make a big difference to maintaining motivation.

REALISE WHEN EXPECTATIONS ARE UNREALISTIC

Assess your own expectations by asking yourself if they are reasonable for others, for example, your best friend.

Expectation:
Unrealistic – I must avoid all treat foods.
Realistic – I can include treat foods sometimes.

REALISE YOU ARE UNIQUE

Striving to be a size or weight you have seen in others but have never been yourself just leaves you overworked and frustrated. Try to enjoy yourself and relax when it comes to eating and exercise.

Expectation:
Pressured – I must be size 10.
Acceptance – A healthy size 14 is OK.

ALLOW YOURSELF TO FEEL DISAPPOINTED

If you didn't achieve what you set out to achieve in a day, allow yourself to feel disappointed. Reassure yourself you are doing the best you can and are making positive changes to your lifestyle and your disappointment will eventually pass.

ACCEPT MISTAKES

Everyone makes mistakes. Learn from them and move on.

ENJOY THE JOURNEY

Being happy only when you achieve a particular goal weight means missing out on a lot of living. Focusing on the present will help you enjoy life every day.

Goal Focus:
Future – I'll feel better if I lose weight.
Present – I'll enjoy today, no matter what my weight is.

BE FLEXIBLE

Allow some flexibility with your goals. You can't predict exactly what will happen so allow the outcome to be a little different to what you had planned. As long as you're heading in the right direction, you'll reach your goals.

Goal:
Rigid – I need to exercise for 1 hour every day.
Flexible – I can manage 4 days of exercise this week.

IMPORTANCE OF TREATS

When trying to lose weight, it's important to allow yourself 'treats' now and then. Building treats into your meal plan helps you stay on track and adds enjoyment to your new eating pattern. Make sure you feel relaxed around food and comfortable with the idea that all foods are acceptable in a balanced and varied eating plan. No food is bad. Aim to eat well 80% of the time and allow 20% for discrepancies. This is a realistic and more sustainable approach to healthy eating.

PRACTICAL WEIGHT LOSS TIPS

- Choose skim or low-fat dairy products.
- Choose low-fat food options where possible.
- Read the nutritional panels on food labels to compare the kilojoules in different foods.
- Increase the vegetable portion of meals.
- Replace sour cream with low-fat natural yoghurt.
- Replace cream with low-fat/light evaporated milk.
- Switch to lemon juice or balsamic vinegar on salads.
- Reduce the oil used when cooking or use non-stick pans.
- Grill or bake meats and fish.
- Increase fruits and vegetables.
- Snack on carrot and celery sticks with salsa.

- Eat meals slowly. Allow time for your brain to register when you are full.
- Ask for entrée-size meals when eating out.
- Choose tomato-based sauces.
- Ask for dressings and sauces on the side.
- Reduce kilojoule intake when drinking alcohol by mixing drinks with low-kilojoule or diet beverages.
- When drinking alcohol, make every second drink non-alcoholic and low in kilojoules such as water or diet soft drinks.
- Use herbs and spices to flavour foods.
- Keep a diary and record everything you eat to help see where you might be going wrong.
- When sugar cravings hit, try eating a small portion of dried fruit.
- Increase your fibre intake with apples, pears, wholegrain cereals, beans, and lentils to feel fuller with lower kilojoules.
- Choose pretzels over potato chips when snacking.
- Never skip a meal and always eat breakfast.

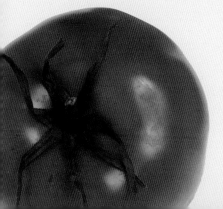

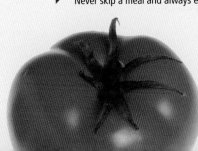

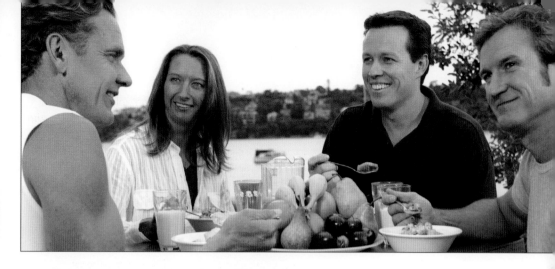

GENETIC, AGE, AND SEX FACTORS

Research suggests there are some people who are more susceptible to becoming overweight or obese than others. Twin, adoption, and family studies have shown genetics play a large role in determining our weight and body shape. For example, twins who are adopted and raised in separate families resemble the body shape and weight of their biological twin more closely than their adopted siblings.

Gender is another important factor in determining our body weight and shape. Women are more efficient than men at storing and conserving body fat. This is an important mechanism for survival of the human race, allowing females to continue their reproductive function in the face of food shortages or famine. Body fat is also stored differently in men and women. Women generally store fat around the hips and thighs, whereas men store fat around the waist.

The fact that men are larger and have greater muscle mass means a man will use more energy than a woman to walk the same distance. For example, an average-sized man will use about 40% more energy than an average-sized woman to walk 1 kilometre. This means most men find it easier to lose weight when they reduce their food intake and start exercising regularly.

Another important factor determining body weight is ageing. Physiological changes with ageing make it easier to gain weight and more difficult to lose it. This could be due to: a reduction in the metabolic rate, reduced lean muscle mass, less physical activity, or increased food intake.

There are also gender differences in the ageing process. Postmenopausal women experience a shift in their body fat from the lower to upper body. These changes mean we need to employ different strategies for reducing body fat at different stages of life.

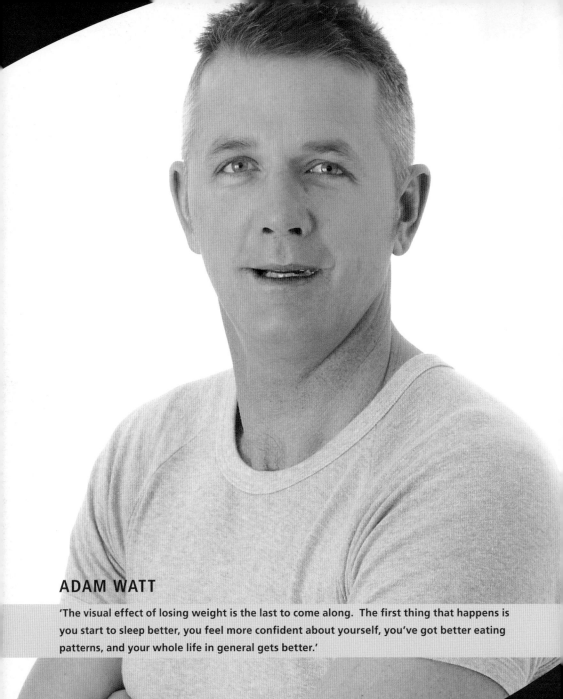

ADAM WATT

'The visual effect of losing weight is the last to come along. The first thing that happens is you start to sleep better, you feel more confident about yourself, you've got better eating patterns, and your whole life in general gets better.'

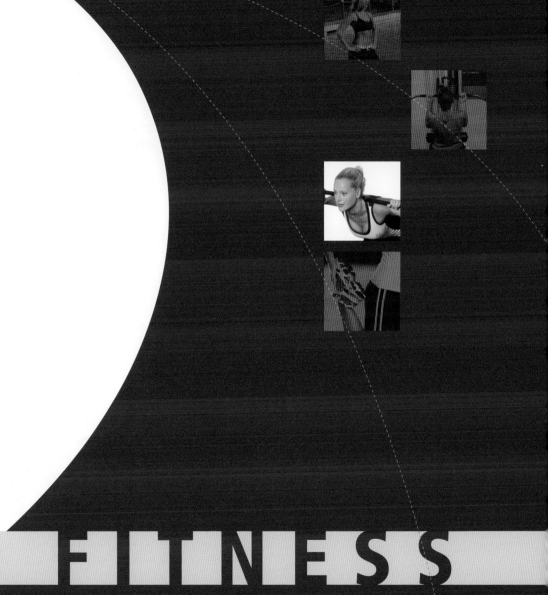

FITNESS

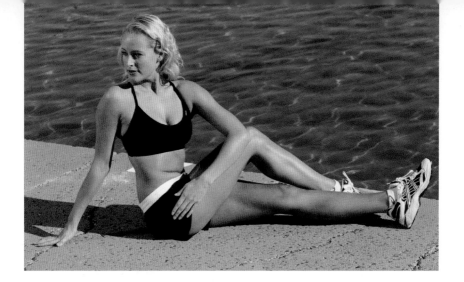

FITNESS TRAINING

Experts in weight loss agree exercise is the best accompaniment to diet when trying to lose body fat.

For a fitness program to be effective, several styles of exercise should be performed, and Fitsmart recommends 3. Stretching is aimed at improving the flexibility of the body's muscle, cardiovascular training burns energy and exercises the heart, and strength training increases the amount of energy burned at rest by increasing the amount of active tissue in the body.

STRETCHING

When we exercise, the muscles are used in ways they are not typically used. This often leads to stiffness and soreness for a few days called delayed onset muscle soreness (DOMS). It is your body's reaction to being trained in new ways. A positive aspect to this soreness is the muscles become stronger as a result. However, as the muscles become stronger, the range of motion of a joint often decreases. Lack of flexibility can be prevented by stretching before and after exercise and will also improve muscle flexibility.

For the muscles to be stretched effectively, they must be warmed and held for a sufficient time period to allow the muscle to relax. We recommend stretches be held at a slight point of discomfort for 30-60 seconds after some form of cardiovascular exercise, after a 5-10 minute warm-up, or at the end of a workout.

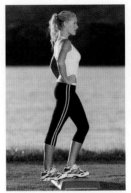

CALVES

Stand on a step with the toes and the ball of 1 foot on the edge. Lower the heel towards the floor without bending the knee. Swap legs and repeat.

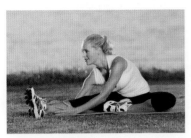

HAMSTRINGS

Sit on the floor and bend 1 knee, keeping the other leg straight. Reach forward with the arms towards the toes.

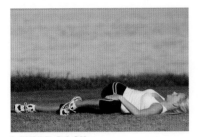

LOWER BACK

Lie on your back with 1 leg straight and the other knee bent to 90 degrees. Keep the shoulders on the ground and drop the bent knee towards the floor on the opposite side. Repeat with other leg.

Advanced: Keep both legs straight.

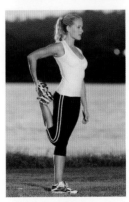

QUADRICEPS

Stand tall and hold 1 ankle from behind and draw it in close, keeping the hips pushed forward.

Advanced: Kneel and place 1 leg forward with the shin vertical. Reach the other leg back behind the body, hold the foot and draw it up. Push the hips forward and lean the torso back.

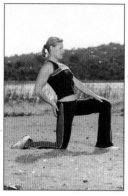

HIP FLEXOR

Kneel, with the right leg forward and the shin vertical. Place the other leg behind with the shin on the ground. Push the hips forward and lean the torso back.

Advanced: Place the right hand on the right hip and reach the left hand up and over to the right.

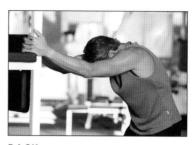

BACK

Grab an immovable object with both arms at chest height and arch the spine away from the hands.

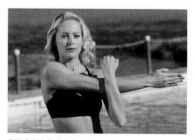

SHOULDERS

Straighten 1 arm and pull it across the front of the body with the other arm pushing the elbow.

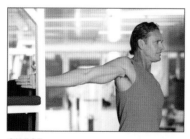

CHEST

Keep the arm straight and place 1 palm on a wall. Turn the body away from the wall, leaving the hand in place.

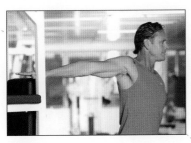

BICEPS

Place the thumb and first finger of 1 hand against a wall. Turn the body away from the wall, leaving the hand in place.

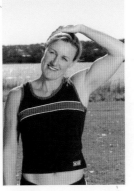

NECK

Place 1 hand on the head and the other hand beside the body. Draw the head to the side and slightly to the front, pulling the other arm down.

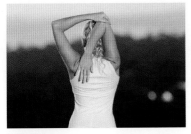

TRICEPS

Reach 1 elbow up to the roof with the hand pointing to the ground. Place the other hand on the elbow and gradually push it down.

CARDIOVASCULAR EXERCISE

Cardiovascular (CV) training is the most effective form of exercise to expend energy and aid weight loss. CV training elevates the heart rate for prolonged periods and causes breathing to increase. It exercises our heart and lungs, and burns fat and carbohydrates. For CV training to be most effective it must involve large muscle groups.

Research has found by improving CV fitness, we reduce the risk of developing certain cancers, cardiovascular disease, diabetes, osteoarthritis, osteoporosis, and obesity. Being aerobically fit also has a positive effect on mental health, energy levels, and aids stability.

Cardiovascular exercise can be performed with or without equipment. A gym can offer equipment specifically designed to improve cardiovascular fitness.

▶ **Stationary bike**
▶ **Treadmill**
▶ **Stepper**
▶ **Rowing machine**
▶ **Cross-trainer machine**

Exercise that doesn't rely on gym equipment.

▶ **Running, walking, cycling**
▶ **Swimming, surfing**
▶ **Rollerblading, skiing**
▶ **Basketball, netball, soccer, football**
▶ **Dancing**
▶ **Martial arts**

There are essentially 2 forms of CV exercise. The first is the continuous approach, where you exercise at a lower intensity for a set period of time without stopping. The second approach is interval training which alternates periods of higher intensity with low intensity exercise.

An example of continuous CV exercise would be going for a brisk walk for 45 minutes without stopping. Interval training would be running for 2 minutes then walking for 2 minutes over a 30-minute period. You could also do interval training on a stationary bike at the gym by adjusting the level of resistance on the bike every few minutes. Interval training is a great way to break up a long session of exercise.

Intensity during CV exercise is based on how quickly your heart is beating, or a percentage of its maximum capacity. You can measure this by taking your pulse for a minute. You can also measure intensity by paying attention to your breath as you exercise.

EASY = just puffing, but able to talk

MODERATE = puffing, talking is laboured

HARD = heavy puffing, unable to talk

To achieve the best results from the CV workouts, you must warm up for around 10 minutes. It is also important to warm down to resting levels after a CV session for around 10 minutes. Both the warm-up and warm-down involve a light form of the CV exercise being performed in the workout.

STRENGTH TRAINING

Strength training is performed using free weights, machine equipment, or with body weight.

Strength training is indispensable in a weight loss exercise program. When anybody diets or restricts the amount of food they are used to eating, the body naturally breaks down its own muscle tissue to help aid weight loss. This constitutes a big part of the weight loss after the first few weeks of dieting. Unfortunately, the loss in muscle tissue also reduces the body's energy burning potential at rest, making weight easy to regain once a normal diet is resumed. Strength training has been shown to reduce the amount of muscle loss when one begins to lose weight from dieting and increase the amount of energy burned at rest by 7-9%. By combining strength training with cardiovascular exercise, you are on the path to effective and healthy fat loss.

Lifting weights has numerous health benefits.

▸ **Increased metabolic rate**
▸ **Increased muscle mass and strength**
▸ **Increased bone mineral density**
▸ **Improved glucose metabolism**
▸ **Improved blood lipid levels**
▸ **Reduced lower back pain**
▸ **Reduced arthritic pain**
▸ **Improved gastrointestinal transit**
▸ **Improved physical function and stability**

WEIGHT SELECTION

For weight-based strength exercises, the size of the weights you use is determined by the point of failure. You should not be able to perform any more repetitions with correct form than the amount stated, e.g., 15-20. If you can do more than the highest number, the weight is too light. If you cannot lift the lowest number, it is too heavy.

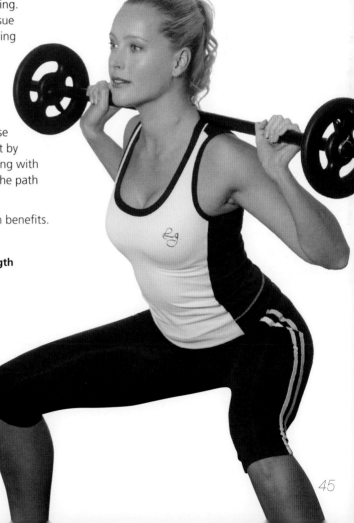

When performing all strength exercises, try to concentrate on exhaling during the lifting part of the movement, and inhaling during the lowering.

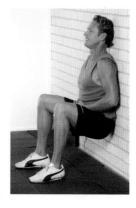

QUADRICEPS:

SKI SQUATS

Step 1: Stand with your back against a wall and position your feet hip-width apart a thigh's distance from the wall.

Step 2: Hold for 15 to 30 seconds, then lower the back 5 centimetres.

Step 3: Repeat Step 2 another 4 times. The last hold should see your thighs below parallel to the floor.

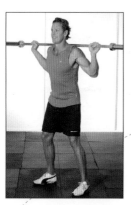
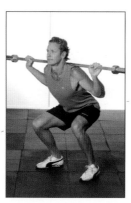

BARBELL SQUATS

Step 1: Stand tall with your feet parallel and wider than shoulder-width apart, and place the barbell on your shoulders.

Step 2: Lower your hips back and down, with the weight on your heels.

Step 3: Pause in the squat position, then rise.

DUMBBELL SQUATS

Step 1: Hold a pair of dumbbells and stand tall with your feet parallel and wider than shoulder-width apart.

Step 2: Lower your hips back and down, with the weight on your heels.

Step 3: Pause in the squat position, then rise.

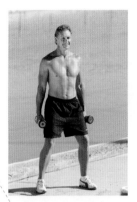 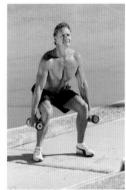

STEP-UPS

Step 1: Stand side on and place 1 foot on a low bench so your thigh is parallel to the floor.

Step 2: Step up on the platform while lifting the knee of your other leg to thigh height.

Step 3: Pause, then step down again.

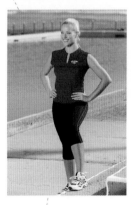 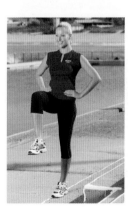

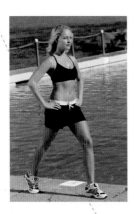 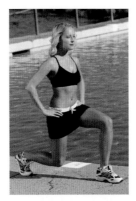

STATIC LUNGES

Step 1: Stand tall and take a large step forward to kneel on the floor.

Step 2: Push on your front heel to rise until your front knee almost locks.

Step 3: Pause, then lower until your knee almost touches the ground. Pause, and repeat.

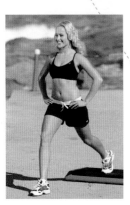 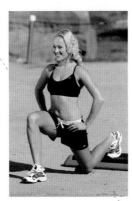

BULGARIAN SQUATS

Step 1: Rest 1 foot on a low bench and step out so your front shin is vertical to the floor.

Step 2: Keep the weight on your heel and lower by pushing your hips back and down.

Step 3: Pause just before your knee touches the ground, then rise.

WIDE SQUATS

Step 1: Stand tall with your feet wider than shoulder-width apart and your toes turned out slightly. Place the bar across your shoulders.

Step 2: Lower your hips back and down, keeping the weight on your heels.

Step 3: Pause in the squat position before your back rounds, then rise.

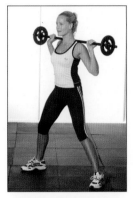 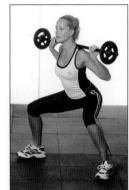

DYNAMIC LUNGES

Step 1: Stand tall with your feet parallel and hip-width apart. Take a large step forward so your front shin is vertical to the floor.

Step 2: Pause and lower slowly.

Step 3: As your knee almost touches the ground, use your heel to spring up and return to standing.

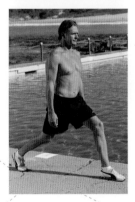 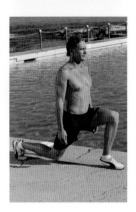

49

HAMSTRINGS, GLUTES, LOWER BACK:

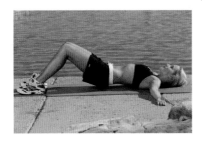
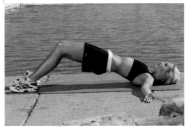

HIP EXTENSIONS

Step 1: Lie on your back with your knees bent to 90 degrees and your feet hip-width apart.

Step 2: Lift your hips until your knees, hips and shoulders are aligned, and squeeze your buttocks together.

Step 3: Pause and lower to starting position.

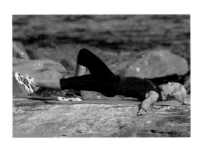
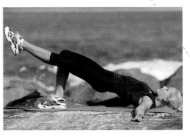

SINGLE LEG HIP EXTENSIONS

Step 1: Lie on your back with 1 knee bent to 90 degrees. Lift your straight leg off the floor.

Step 2: Lift your hips until your knees, hips and shoulders are aligned, and both thighs are together. Squeeze your glutes.

Step 3: Lower and pause just before your buttocks and leg touch the ground, then repeat.

MODIFIED LEG CURLS

Step 1: Hook both legs under the knee support pads of a machine, such as a lat pulldown.

Step 2: Lean your torso forward, moving only from your knees.

Step 3: Lower as far as possible before your hips bend. Pause, and return to starting position.

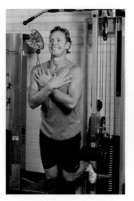 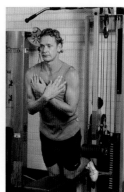

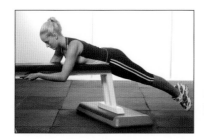 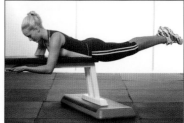

REVERSE BACK EXTENSIONS

Step 1: Lie face down on a bench and position your hips so they are just off the end with your feet on the floor. Keep your feet together and your legs straight with a slight bend in your knees.

Step 2: Lift your legs up so they are parallel to the floor and your feet reach the same height as the hips.

Step 3: Pause in the top position, then lower until the toes almost touch the ground.

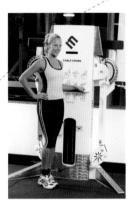
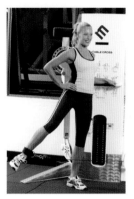

CABLE SINGLE LEG ABDUCTIONS

Step 1: Attach the strap of a low cable machine to your ankle, take 2 steps away from the base of the pulley system and stand side on. Keep your torso upright and hold the arm support.

Step 2: Lift your strapped leg out to the side as high as possible before your torso begins to lean.

Step 3: Pause, then return to starting position.

ROMANIAN DEADLIFTS

Step 1: Stand tall with your knees slightly bent and your feet hip-width apart and parallel. With your hands shoulder-width apart, rest the bar on your thighs, keeping the weight on your heels.

Step 2: Push the buttocks back and bend forward from the hips, keeping the bar in contact with the thighs.

Step 3: Pause before your spine rounds, squeeze your buttocks, then rise.

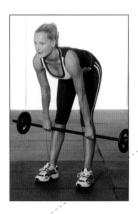

GOOD MORNINGS

Step 1: Stand tall with the bar on your shoulders, your knees slightly bent, and your feet hip-width apart and parallel.

Step 2: Push your buttocks back and bow forward from the hips, keeping the weight on your heels.

Step 3: Pause before the spine rounds, squeeze your buttocks, and return to starting position.

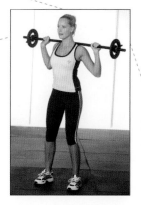 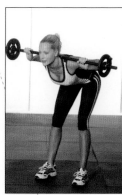

DUMBBELL ROMANIAN DEADLIFTS

Step 1: Hold a pair of dumbbells with your knees slightly bent and feet hip-width apart and parallel.

Step 2: Push your buttocks back and bow forward from your hips, keeping the dumbbells in contact with your thighs and the weight on your heels.

Step 3: Pause before the spine rounds, squeeze your buttocks, and return to starting position.

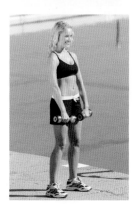 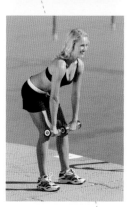

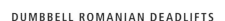

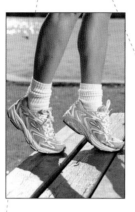

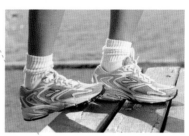

CALVES:

SINGLE LEG STANDING CALF RAISE

Step 1: Stand tall with the toes of 1 leg on the edge of a step. Keep your knees slightly bent.

Step 2: Push on your toes to lift your heel high.

Step 3: Pause, then lower past the level of the step, and repeat.

BENT KNEE CALF RAISE

Step 1: Sit on a bench and place your toes on a low step with the weight over your thighs.

Step 2: Push on the tips of your toes to lift your heels.

Step 3: Pause, then return to starting position.

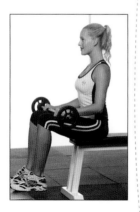

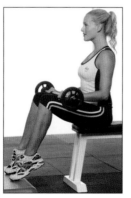

CHEST:

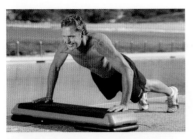 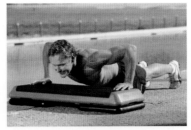

HANDS ELEVATED PUSH-UPS

Step 1: Set the push-up position with your hands elevated on a step or bench.

Step 2: Lower your body, bending from the elbows and keeping the torso straight.

Step 3: Pause when your chest reaches a fist's distance from the step, then push back to starting position.

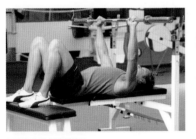 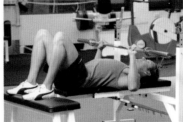

BENCH PRESS

Step 1: Lie on a bench press station, with your knees bent and your feet flat on the bench. Grip the bar wider than shoulder-width apart.

Step 1: Unrack the bar and hold it at arm's length over your lower chest.

Step 3: Lower the bar until it almost touches your lower chest, pause, then push the bar back to starting position.

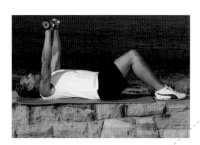 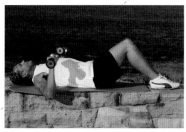

DUMBBELL BENCH PRESS

Step 1: Lie on a bench with your knees bent and your feet flat. Hold the dumbbells so they are touching above your lower chest.

Step 2: Lower the dumbbells down and out in an upside-down V pattern until your hands are in line with your lower chest.

Step 3: Pause, then push back to starting position.

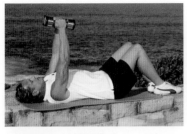
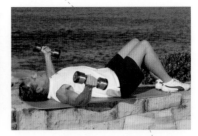

DUMBBELL FLYES

Step 1: Lie on a bench and hold the dumbbells so they face each other.

Step 2: Lower your arms away from your body to the side.

Step 3: Pause when your arms reach chest level, then push back to starting position.

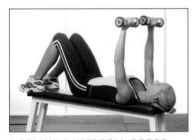
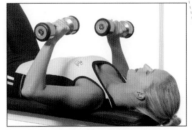

DECLINE DUMBBELL PRESS

Step 1: Lie on a decline bench with your head at the lowest end, your knees bent and your feet flat.

Step 2: Lower the dumbbells down and out in an upside-down V pattern until your hands are in line with your lower chest.

Step 3: Pause, then push back to starting position.

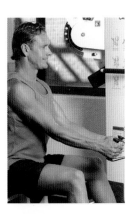
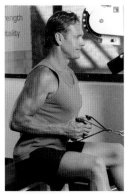

MIDDLE/UPPER BACK:

SEATED ROW

Step 1: In the seated position, grip the seated row bar.

Step 2: Pull your elbows back and into your body.

Step 3: Pause when the bar reaches your lower abdominals, then return to starting position.

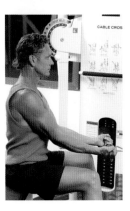
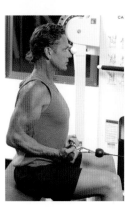

SEATED ROW UNDERHAND GRIP

Step 1: In the seated position, grip the seated row bar with an underhand grip.

Step 2: Pull your elbows back and into the body.

Step 3: Pause when the bar reaches your lower abdominals, then return to starting position.

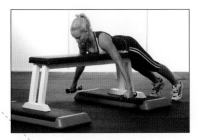 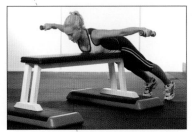

PRONE FLYES

Step 1: Lie face down on a bench with your hips just off the end, your feet hip-width apart, and your toes on the floor.

Step 2: Hold the dumbbells, and lift your arms out to the side of your chest.

Step 3: When your arms reach shoulder level, squeeze the shoulder blades together, pause, then return to starting position.

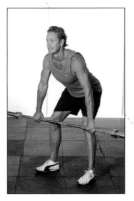 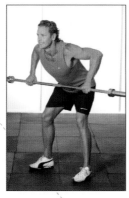

BENT OVER ROWS

Step 1: Stand with your knees slightly bent and your feet hip-width apart and parallel. Hold a bar wider than shoulder-width apart, resting it on the thighs. Push your buttocks back and bend from your hips.

Step 2: Pull your elbows up to the roof, keeping them close to your body.

Step 3: When the bar reaches the torso, pause, then return to starting position.

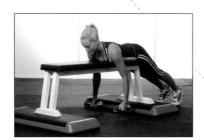 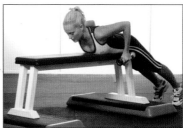

DUMBBELL ROWS

Step 1: Lie face down on a bench with your hips just off the end, your feet hip-width apart, and your toes on the floor.

Step 2: Hold the dumbbells, and pull your elbows up close to the body, while drawing your shoulder blades together and down.

Step 3: When your hands reach your torso, pause, then return to starting position.

MIDDLE/LOWER BACK:

LAT PULLDOWN WIDE GRIP

Step 1: Hold a lat pulldown bar wider than shoulder-width apart.

Step 2: Lean your torso back slightly and pull your elbows down towards your torso.

Step 3: Pause when the bar reaches mouth height, then return to starting position.

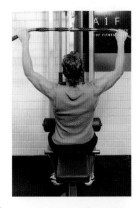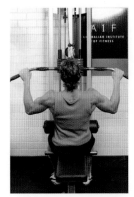

LAT PULLDOWN NARROW GRIP

Step 1: Hold a narrow grip lat pulldown device.

Step 2: Lean your torso back slightly and pull your elbows down towards your torso.

Step 3: Pause when your hands reach reaches mouth height, then return to starting position.

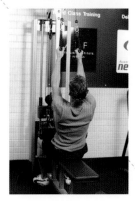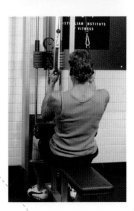

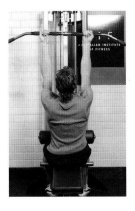 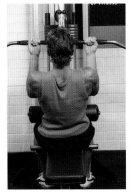

LAT PULLDOWN UNDERHAND GRIP

Step 1: Hold a lat pulldown bar shoulder-width apart with your palms facing you.

Step 2: Lean your torso back slightly and pull your elbows down towards your torso.

Step 3: Pause when the bar reaches mouth height, then return to starting position.

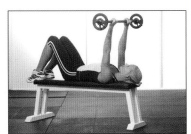 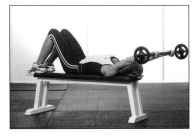

BARBELL PULLOVERS

Step 1: Lie on a bench with your knees bent and your feet up. Hold the barbell above your chest with your hands shoulder-width apart.

Step 2: Lower the barbell away from your body towards your head.

Step 3: Pause when your arms reach your ears, then return to starting position.

SHOULDERS:

LATERAL RAISE

Step 1: Stand tall and hold a pair of dumbbells beside your thighs.

Step 2: Lift your arms out to the side with your hands in the same line as your shoulders.

Step 3: When your arms are parallel to the floor, pause, then return to starting position.

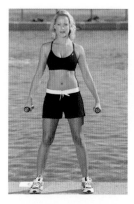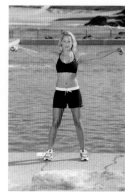

FRONTAL RAISE

Step 1: Stand tall and hold a pair of dumbbells just above the knees.

Step 2: Lift your arms up keeping your hands in line with your shoulders.

Step 3: When your arms are parallel to the floor, pause, then return to starting position.

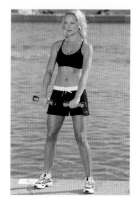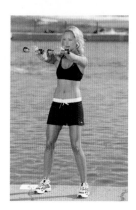

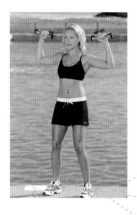
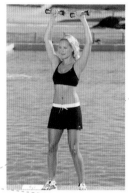

DUMBBELL SHOULDER PRESS

Step 1: Stand tall and hold a pair of dumbbells. Position the arms to create a 90 degree angle in your elbow and shoulder joints. Keep your hands facing forward.

Step 2: Push both hands upwards in a pyramid shape.

Step 3: When the dumbbells almost touch overhead, pause, then lower to starting position.

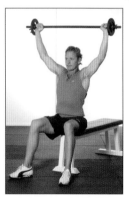
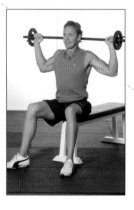

BARBELL SHOULDER PRESS

Step 1: Sit on the end of a bench and hold the barbell much wider than shoulder-width apart.

Step 2: Lower the barbell behind the neck, keeping your wrists straight and elbows back.

Step 3: Pause when the barbell reaches ear height, then push up to starting position.

BICEPS:

BARBELL CURLS

Step 1: Stand tall and hold a barbell with hands shoulder-width apart.

Step 2: Curl up to shoulder height, keeping your elbows in.

Step 3: Pause, then lower to starting position.

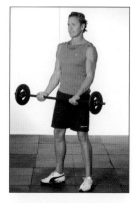 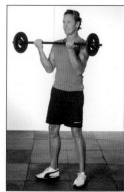

ZOTTMAN CURLS

Step 1: Stand tall and hold a pair of dumbbells with your palms facing up.

Step 2: Lift the dumbbells to shoulder height, pause, then face your palms down.

Step 3: Lower the dumbbells back to starting position, pause, then face your palms up.

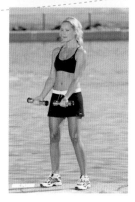 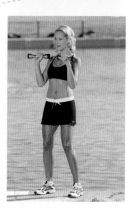

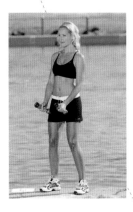 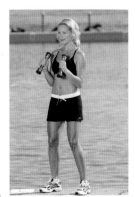

HAMMER CURLS

Step 1: Stand tall and hold a pair of dumbbells with the palms facing up.

Step 2: Curl the dumbbells up to shoulder height.

Step 3: Pause, then lower to starting position.

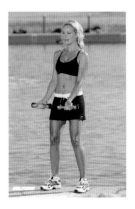 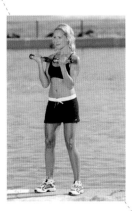

DUMBBELL CURLS

Step 1: Stand tall and hold a pair of dumbbells to face each other.

Step 2: Curl the dumbbells up to shoulder height.

Step 3: Pause, then lower to starting position.

REVERSE GRIP DUMBBELL CURLS

Step 1: Stand tall and hold a pair of dumbbells with the palms facing down.

Step 2: Curl the dumbbells up to shoulder height.

Step 3: Pause, then lower to starting position.

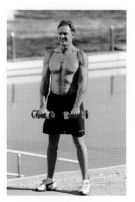 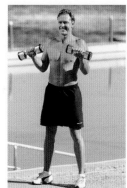

DUMBBELL CURLS WITH TWIST

Step 1: Stand tall and hold a pair of dumbbells to face each other.

Step 2: As you curl the dumbbells up to shoulder height, twist your hands so your palms face up.

Step 3: Pause, then lower the same way as they were lifted.

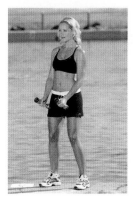 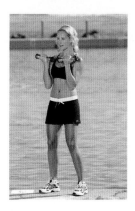

TRICEPS:

TRICEP PUSHDOWNS

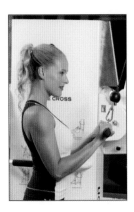
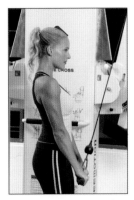

Step 1: Stand tall and grip the bar shoulder-width apart with your palms facing down.

Step 2: Push the bar down until your elbows are straightened, but not locked.

Step 3: Pause, then return to starting position.

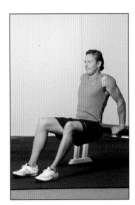
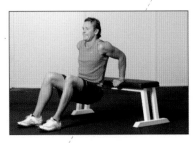

DIPS

Step 1: Sit on the side of a bench with your hands shoulder-width apart on the edge and your feet forward.

Step 2: Lower your hips to the floor and pause when your elbows reach 90 degrees.

Step 3: Push on the bench to straighten your arms and return to starting position.

OVERHEAD TRICEP EXTENSIONS

Step 1: Grip 1 dumbbell with both hands at arm's distance above the head.

Step 2: Lower the dumbbell down to the back of your head, keeping your elbows in.

Step 3: Pause when the dumbbell reaches your neck, then return to starting position.

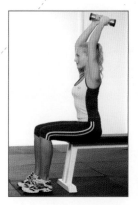 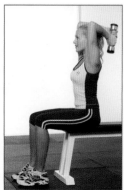

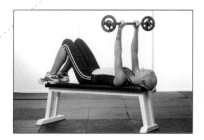 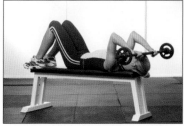

LYING TRICEP EXTENSIONS

Step 1: Lie on a bench with your knees bent and your feet flat, and hold the bar at arm's length over your head.

Step 2: Lower the bar until it almost touches the start of your hairline.

Step 3: Pause, then push the bar back to starting position.

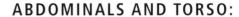

ABDOMINALS AND TORSO:

FRONT BRIDGE

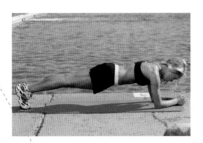

Step 1: Lie face down, with your elbows underneath the shoulders and your forearms parallel.

Step 2: Lift your hips and balance your weight between your toes and elbows.

Step 3: Tighten your abdominals and maintain constant breathing. Keep your back flat and your torso parallel to the floor. Hold for as long as possible.

Beginners: Perform this exercise by creating the bridge between your elbows and knees.

SIDE BRIDGE

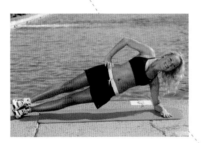

Step 1: Lie on your side and position your elbow under your shoulder. Rest your other arm on your body.

Step 2: Lift your hips so your torso aligns with your legs and head, and your weight is balanced between your elbow and feet.

Step 3: Tighten your abdominals and maintain constant breathing. Hold for as long as possible.

Beginners: Perform this exercise by creating the bridge between your elbows and knees.

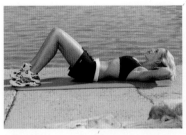 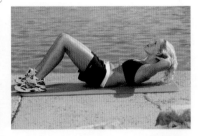

SIT-UPS

Step 1: Lie on the floor with your knees bent and your hands behind your head.

Step 2: Lift your upper back off the floor several centimetres.

Step 3: Pause, then return to starting position.

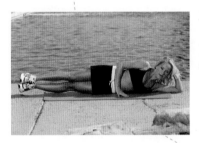 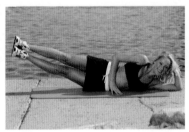

SIDE LEG RAISE

Step 1: Lie on your side, and place one hand behind your head and the other on the floor.

Step 2: Lift both legs as high as possible.

Step 3: Pause, then return to starting position.

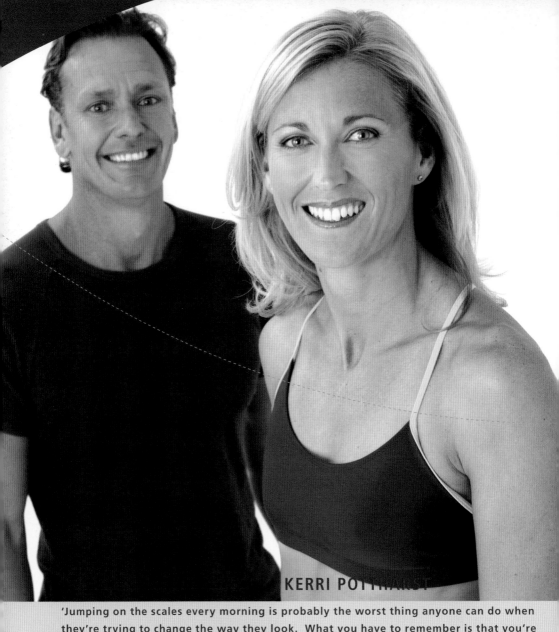

KERRI POTTHARST

'Jumping on the scales every morning is probably the worst thing anyone can do when they're trying to change the way they look. What you have to remember is that you're doing this not just to look better but to feel better, too.'

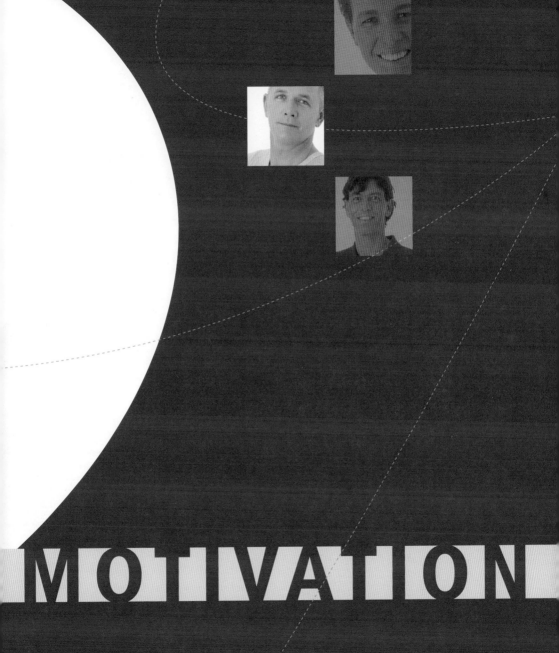

MOTIVATION

how the stars
stay motivated

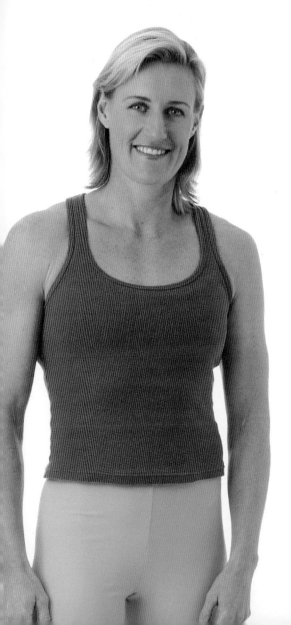

We can't achieve anything in life without having goals. It's what's going to get you out on a rainy day when you don't feel like getting out of bed and going for that walk or jog or going to the gym. That's what a goal is.

Guy Leech

When things aren't going right, that is the time you have to see the big picture. Maybe it's a year down the track that you want to lose 10kg and this week you haven't lost anything or you might have even put on weight. Don't worry about that; all of us have had hurdles and I can tell you all of us have had to get through them.

Shelley Oates Wilding

MOTIVATION TIPS

- ▸ Vary exercise routines and try different sports.
- ▸ Set achievable goals and keep it in perspective.
- ▸ Work fitness into social activities.
- ▸ When exercising, focus on different aspects of movement to keep brain active.
- ▸ Keep focus of the long-term goal.

To maintain motivation you also have to set goals. Whether it's that week, that month, or in six months, you have to put your training methods around where your goal should be. Whether you go to the gym or you go mountain biking, just try to keep a lot of the fitness things fun. That way, your motivation will always stay up there.

Sandon Stolle

The good thing is if you start being active, you'll like to be active all the time. I've found it usually gets boring as a constant day-to-day thing. If you mix it up and have several different days a week, where you change each day and keep up with that variety, it all starts coming together. Your body starts loving it and you just don't want to miss out on it, on that daily process.

Tom Carroll

You just have to change things. If surfing gets boring, I go to another beach, or I go surfing with friends and just break it up a bit. I'll add some variety to it—try different boards, get a new board, try an old single fin, just something that challenges me. That's what keeps it exciting. Once you stop being challenged, that's when it starts to get boring.

Layne Beachley

When you're an elite athlete, all you're doing is training. The challenge for me was when I finished formal competition to fit exercise into my day. I've got a daughter and have to look after her, drop her to school, and do everything else so I fit exercise into my daily routine. Make it a social occasion. Get out there with some mates and do a run. Or go and play some tennis or squash.

Steven Lee

When I was doing Olympic-distance swimming training, I'd try to focus on different aspects of what I was doing, whether it would be times for every 50m or times for my 100m, or thinking about my stroke, just to keep the brain mentally active. Now, I try doing different sporting activities, and mix up my weekly routines. Even though 9 times out of 10 you actually are doing exactly the same thing, it only takes a small change, just a little bit of a difference in your routine, to keep you excited about what you're doing.

Kieren Perkins

Fitting everything into the day is not difficult at all. You just have to be structured. You have to set up your schedule so that you can put time away for exercise. So, even if it just takes 30 minutes a day to do what you have to do to feel good, that's all it takes. Look, if you can't afford 30 minutes a day, you can't afford to be healthy.

Greg Welch

The way I work to achieve a goal is I set a 1-week block at a time. One week out, I sit down on the Sunday and have a look at the Monday to Sunday program, and that's the way I discipline myself. I say, 'OK, I've got these programs to do. I've got to do this, this week. If I don't do that, I'll have to make up for it.' I promote myself that way.

Adam Watt

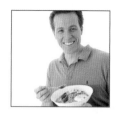

Keeping yourself motivated can be difficult. You're not alone if you have bad days, go off track, or lose sight of the big picture.

Here's a sample of questions from our Internet Fitsmart users and motivating tips from our champion athletes. Believe it or not, they go through the same feelings of doubt, lack of motivation, and time constraints as the rest of us. And they've worked through all of these negative feelings and come out on top.

Problem:

I just can't seem to motivate myself. It just seems like if it's not one thing stopping me from following the plan it's another. What can I do to overcome these obstacles?

Response:

First set your goals and then set a date for your goals! If you keep an event in mind you want to be fit for this will help get you motivated little by little each day.

Remember, this is all about lifestyle, so there will always be easy and hard times. Even if you only have some good meals, and do a little bit of exercise now and then, it's better than nothing! And when life gets easier, you can do more and try to make up for it. Remember, it definitely gets easier with time.

Guy Leech

Problem:

I'm in my third week now and I'm determined to make this a better week than last week! I ate too much and did very little exercise. I have stayed the same weight as the week before, which is better than putting any weight on I suppose, but it's very frustrating.

Response:

Everybody is unique and the way their body adjusts to a healthier eating pattern and increased exercise will differ from person to person. Concentrate on the measurements as your scale weight can fluctuate a great deal even during the course of a day.

Keep reminding yourself everything you do (or don't do) has an effect. Each time you're tempted by food, ask yourself if you also want the extra exercise that goes with it. Once you start thinking about the entire process of food and your body, you'll be more focused on staying on track. But most of all, don't panic. If you do have a bad day or a bad week, then look forward, focus on tomorrow, and start afresh.

Kieren Perkins

Problem:

I really enjoy walking, but some weeks I don't walk much at all because it's so hot where I live. I exercise with my baby daughter by pushing her in the pram and I feel a bit guilty taking her out in the heat. And now I'm feeling lazy and lack the motivation to get going again.

Response:

Maybe try walking early in the morning around sunrise when the sun has no sting in it. You might find it's a really good way to start the day as well. Swimming is also a great one for warm weather—great exercise and a great way to cool off.

Otherwise, you may want to look at getting an exercise bike or doing some aerobic exercise in the house so you can still keep up the activity on days you don't want to venture outside.

Basically, it all comes down to planning. Exercise doesn't just happen—it has to be scheduled into your week. Treat it like everything else you have to do—like washing, shopping, picking up the kids, or going out. Use your diary and be true to it.

We can always find an excuse not to exercise—even champion athletes. Lacking motivation is only natural at some stage of dieting and exercising. Focus on how good you'll feel after it and how at the end of the day when you have made the effort you'll feel proud and motivated.

Adam Watt

Problem:

My husband isn't as worried about his weight as I am. He brings home some alcohol and junk food which he knows I'm trying to avoid and in return he says, 'I'm a bad influence, aren't I?'

I've been trying to lose weight for 5 years and I lose a bit and then put a heap on. Now that I have some motivation to exercise, I feel as though he's dragging me down.

Response:

It can be really tough trying to make a major lifestyle change on your own, especially when you're living with a 'bad influence'. The important thing is not to give up or let the other person be the reason you give up. You are doing this for you and hopefully, once he sees all your hard work, he will come around.

If you're really struggling with his bad influences, then try distracting yourself. When he has something you might be tempted by, go and do something else in another room. If you really find yourself crumbling, then try to limit yourself to having just half of the treat. It's all about compromise, and the sooner you get into that habit the easier you'll find it is making this lifestyle change.

Set a goal to achieve and promise yourself that whatever it takes you will achieve it. Focus on healthy eating and living, rather than just weight loss, and you'll feel a whole lot more positive and motivated.

Shelley Oates Wilding

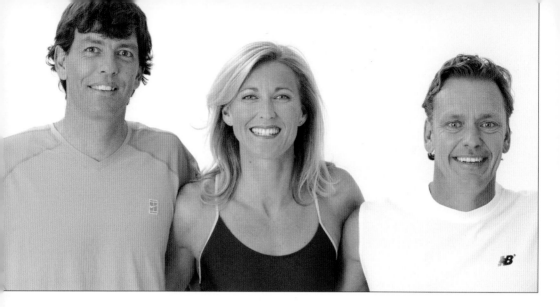

Problem:

I am a working mother with two kids. How do I fit in any sort of exercise routine into my busy schedule?

Response:

This is where support comes in. If you have a close relation or friend, ask for help so that you can get to the gym or go for a swim, or whatever it is you enjoy. It's time consuming being superwoman, but try to set aside time to do an early-morning walk (just 20 minutes or so) or to do some strength exercises at home. Take the kids to the park and kick around a soccer ball, or play chasey or catch on weekends. If they're little, put them in a pram and walk, or, if they're a bit older, get them to ride their bikes while you walk. Even just put some music on and dance in the living room—and let the kids join in!

Sometimes just being more active rather than doing full-on workouts is easier to cope with.

The best thing about involving your kids in your exercise program is that you'll be setting a great example for them. They'll see exercise as a fun thing, not something to dread, and you'll be doing them a huge favour in terms of a healthy lifestyle.

A handy hint for busy mums trying to adhere to the meal plans is to choose meals that you can make in bulk and freeze. That way, on the really hairy days, you only have to thaw something out and add to it. It usually doesn't take any longer to cook double or triple quantities than it does to prepare a single serve, and this way you won't be cooking every night.

Kerri Pottharst

MOTIVATIONAL TIPS

▶ *Focus on centimetres not kilograms.* Your body is being reshaped. Shift your focus from weight to giving yourself credit for the behaviour and attitude changes that have brought you this far.

▶ *Take it one step at a time.* If you've been unable to resist the urge to overeat, or haven't done any exercise one week, then look for small ways to reduce your food intake for the next week and plan your week around your exercise days.

▶ *Use your family.* Many people have found success by involving their family in their diet and exercise routines. Once you show them you are serious about losing weight, you can draw a huge amount of support.

▶ *Don't let your program get boring.* If you're losing interest, it's time to change things around. Find a friend with similar fitness levels to join you. Or go to the park, or the beach, or even just change the time of day you exercise.

▶ *Make an appointment with yourself.* If you're finding lack of time is inhibiting you, you need to make the time. Make exercise a priority and schedule the time in your diary on the days you choose to exercise—and don't cross it out!

▶ *Keep focused on your goals.* Think about all the positive aspects that will come into your life if you achieve the goals you set for yourself. Make sure they're written down where you see them every day. And most importantly, reiterate these goals to yourself, at least 3 times a week.

▶ *Think '80/20'.* Stay on target 80% of the time and 20% of the time relax and enjoy the odd treat. Don't overdo it, but do build in some of the foods you've been missing, with the exception of foods that have addictive qualities, or the foods that may trigger uncontrolled overeating.

▶ *Think like a winner.* Negative self-talk, to yourself or others, tends to exaggerate the gravity of a situation and leads to feelings of despair. Replace negative messages with realistic, positive affirmations such as, 'This is tough, but it's not the end of the world—I'll survive, I can do it.'

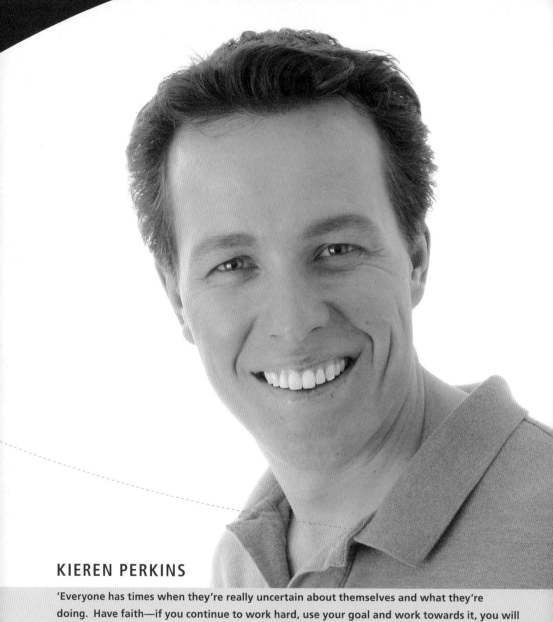

KIEREN PERKINS

'Everyone has times when they're really uncertain about themselves and what they're doing. Have faith—if you continue to work hard, use your goal and work towards it, you will eventually get there.'

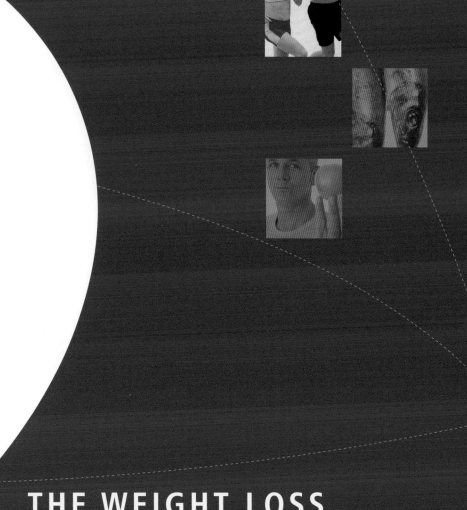

THE WEIGHT LOSS
PROGRAM

PLAN A-MAKE A START

This plan is all about embracing a healthy lifestyle. The following 8 weeks will involve learning about food and focusing on changing your eating and exercise habits gradually. Instead of a strict diet, each week you will have a list of things to do. At the end of the week, tick off those you have achieved and keep doing them. If there are things you haven't achieved, add them to your list for the next week. The fitness program allows you to choose a type of cardio activity you enjoy, plus some strengthening exercises. Once you have completed the 8 weeks, you can continue your new eating habits and exercise program, or, if you find your weight loss is slowing down, move to Plan B or C for a more specific, kilojoule-controlled plan with more exercise.

weeks 1 & 2

FOOD PROGRAM

WEEK 1 – FOCUS ON FAT

The aim this week is to reduce the amount of fat in your diet, particularly saturated fats. Read nutrition information on packaged products and choose those lowest in saturated fats. Refer to pages 22 and 23.

Week 1 checklist

▸ **Trim the fat from meat before you cook it.**

▸ **For all recipes, use a maximum of 1 tablespoon of oil for every 2 servings. Make sure it is monounsaturated or polyunsaturated oil e.g., peanut, sunflower, olive, canola, or safflower.**

▸ **Remove the skin off chicken before you cook it.**

▸ **Avoid deep-fried foods.**

▸ **Use margarine and high-fat spreads sparingly.**

▸ **Switch to low-fat dairy products.**

▸ **Replace cream with low-fat natural yoghurt or reduced-fat evaporated milk.**

▸ **Limit takeaway meals to once a week.**

▸ **Limit biscuits, cakes, and pastries to once a week.**

▸ **Write down what you eat and calculate how many grams of fat you have in a day. Aim for 60-80g for men, and 40-60g for women.**

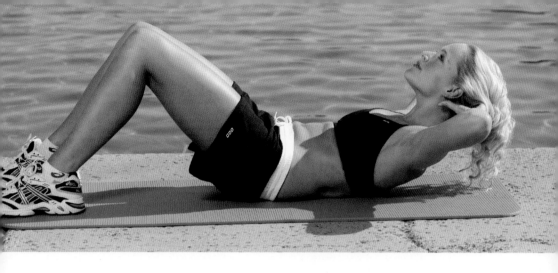

WEEK 2 – MANAGE PORTIONS

This week the focus is on how much you eat. Too much of anything will make it harder to lose weight. Read the nutrition panels on foods you buy and compare kilojoule values.

Week 2 checklist

▶ **Aim for your dinner plate to contain half vegetables or salad, half a combination of meat, fish or alternatives, and starchy foods such as rice, pasta, potato, or bread.**

▶ **Ask for small or regular sizes.**

▶ **At restaurants, have two entrées rather than an entrée and a main course.**

▶ **Buy bread cut into thin slices.**

▶ **Serve meals on smaller dishes.**

▶ **Eat a third less than you normally would.**

FITNESS PROGRAM

Total days per week: 5
Cardio training days: 3
Strength training days: 2
Total time: 3-4 hours

The emphasis for this program is continuous cardiovascular sessions such as walking plus some basic strength training exercises.

For all strength training (ST) exercises during Week 1 to Week 4, you should aim for 2 sets of 15-20 repetitions, using a 3 second lowering speed, 1 second pause, and a 3 second lifting speed. These are best performed with only a 60 second rest between sets.

The order that the strength exercises are performed is very important, so follow the same order as they are noted in the program.

All cardio sessions require continuous, easy to moderate exercise that increases the heart rate and breathing.

MON

week 1
CV: 35-40mins

MON

week 2
CV: 40-45mins

TUE

ST: 2 sets of 15-20 reps

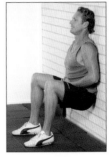

1 Ski squats

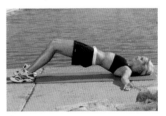

2 Hip extensions

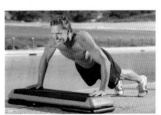

3 Hands elevated push-ups

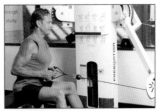

4 Seated row

rest day

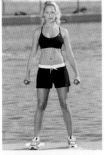 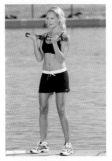

5 Lateral rise   **6** Dumbbell curls

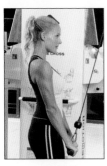

7 Tricep pushdowns

THU

week 1
CV: 30-35mins

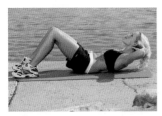

8 Sit-ups

THU

week 2
CV: 35-40mins

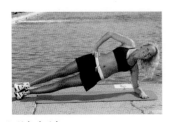

9 Side bridge

ST: 2 sets of 15-20 reps

rest day

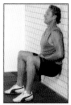

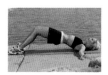

1 Ski squats   **2** Hip extensions

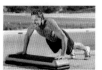

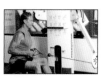

3 Hands elevated push ups   **4** Seated row

SUN

week 1
CV: 30mins

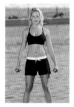

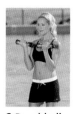

5 Lateral raise   **6** Dumbbell curls

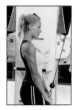

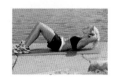

8 Sit-ups

7 Tricep pushdowns

SUN

week 2
CV: 40mins

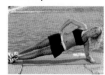

9 Side bridge

weeks 3 & 4

FOOD PROGRAM

WEEK 3 – FOCUS ON REGULAR EATING

Many people think skipping meals is beneficial when trying to lose weight. However, research has shown constantly skipping breakfast can result in a 2.5kg weight increase in a year! Eating regularly throughout the day helps to keep energy levels up, controls appetite, and reduces the risk of overeating.

Week 3 checklist

▸ **Start the day with breakfast. Set your alarm 15 minutes earlier to have time to enjoy your meal. If you aren't hungry in the mornings, try eating less the night before, or waiting for an hour after you get up.**

▸ **Eat healthy snacks to manage your appetite. A piece of fruit or a handful of unsalted nuts between meals can help you eat less at the next meal.**

▸ **Take your lunch to work or keep ready-to-eat foods at work—low kilojoule long-life soups, cans of tuna or baked beans, wholegrain crackers, or low-fat two-minute noodles.**

▸ **Don't go longer than 3-5 hours without a healthy drink or snack to take the edge off your hunger.**

WEEK 4 – EAT FRUIT AND VEG

The high fibre in fruits and vegetables will help satisfy your appetite. Also, since most vegetables are low in kilojoules, eating higher proportions of vegetables as part of your meal will mean you will be eating fewer kilojoules. Remember, starchy vegetables are higher in kilojoules and should be limited to 1 serving a day. These include potato, sweet potato, parsnip, corn, dried beans, and lentils.

Week 4 checklist

▸ **Eat 2 pieces of fruit each day.**

▸ **Eat at least 2½ cups of vegetables each day (excluding potatoes).**

▸ **Only eat potatoes whole, boiled, or roasted without added oil.**

▸ **Avoid fruit juice and eat whole fruit instead.**

▸ **Choose canned fruit in natural juice and drain juice before eating.**

▸ **If using canned vegetables, drain, and rinse before use.**

▸ **Eat fruit and/or vegetables at each meal.**

week 3
CV: 40-45mins

MON

week 4
CV: 45-50mins

ST: 2 sets of 15-20 reps

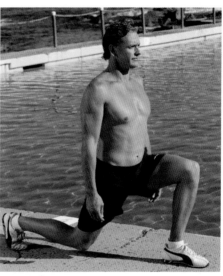

1 Static lunges

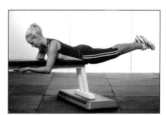

2 Reverse back extensions

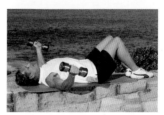

3 Dumbbell flyes

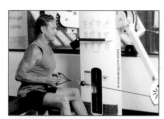

4 Seated row

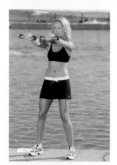

5 Frontal raise

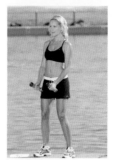

6 Hammer curls

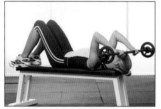

7 Lying tricep extensions

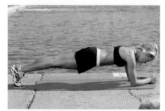

8 Front bridge

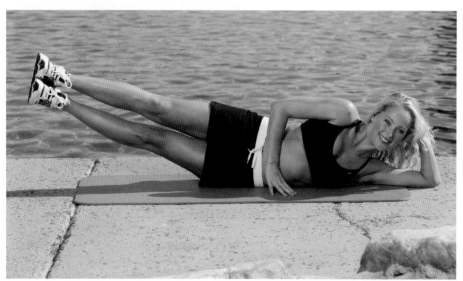

9 Side leg raise

WED

rest day

THU

week 3
CV: 35-40mins

THU

week 4
CV: 40-45mins

FRI

ST: 2 sets of 15-20 reps

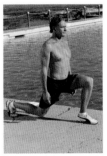

1 Static lunges

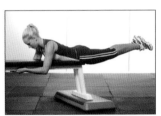

2 Reverse back extensions

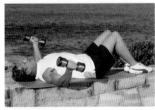

3 Dumbbell flyes

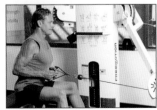

4 Seated row

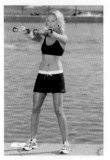
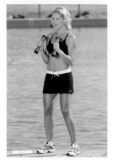

5 Frontal raise   **6** Hammer curls

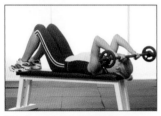

7 Lying tricep extensions

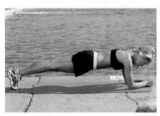

8 Front bridge

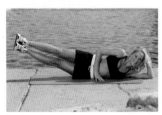

9 Side leg raise

SAT

rest day

SUN

week 3
CV: 30mins

SUN

week 4
CV: 50mins

weeks 5 & 6

FOOD PROGRAM

WEEK 5 – READ LABELS

This week you'll be looking carefully at food labels. The information can tell you a lot about what you are eating and how it will contribute to your daily fat, kilojoule, and nutrient intake. Be wary of foods with 'light' on the label—this doesn't always mean reduced kilojoules or fat. The term 'light' or 'lite' can be used by manufacturers to describe the weight and colour of the food. Also watch for 'fat free' or '99% fat free' as they may still be high in kilojoules.

Read the nutrition information in the per 100g column. If you know how you will be eating and want to know exactly how many kilojoules, grams of fat, or other nutrients you'll be consuming, look at the per serving information. However, note the serving quantity, as it may differ to the amount you actually eat. For example, some yoghurt manufacturers call a serving 100g, when most people actually eat 200g in a serving.

Week 5 checklist

▶ **Compare 'light' or 'fat free' foods with full fat alternatives and note the difference in kilojoules.**

▶ **Choose foods with less than 3g saturated fat per 100g.**

▶ **Choose foods with added sugar with less than 10g sugar per 100g.**

▶ **Choose bread and cereals with more than 3g fibre per serve.**

▶ **Look for low-salt foods with less than 120mg sodium per 100g.**

WEEK 6 – MONITOR FLUIDS

This week it's time to focus on fluids, and in particular, alcohol. Alcohol contains almost as many kilojoules on a gram for gram basis as fat. This means a few glasses of wine or a couple of beers after work will significantly contribute to your daily kilojoule intake. When trying to lose weight the best idea is to minimise your alcohol intake and keep it to special occasions or weekends only.

Other fluids can also significantly add to your daily total kilojoule intake. For example, a 250ml glass of orange juice has 80% more kilojoules than a medium orange and none of the fibre that's found in the whole fruit.

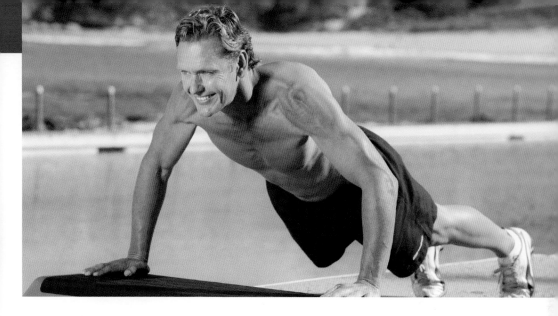

Week 6 checklist

- ▶ **Drink alcohol no more than 2 times a week.**
- ▶ **Set yourself limits when you do drink. For women, no more than 2 standard drinks and for men, no more than 4.**
- ▶ **If going out, limit the time period in which you will drink alcohol, e.g., between 7 and 10pm.**
- ▶ **Reduce the total amount of alcohol you drink by doing the following:**
- ▶ **Drink light beer instead of regular.**
- ▶ **Mix half wine with half soda water.**
- ▶ **Mix spirits with diet soft drinks.**
- ▶ **Have a glass of water or diet soft drink between alcoholic drinks.**
- ▶ **Drink 8 glasses of fluid each day—this includes water (mostly), diet soft drinks, diet cordials, tea, coffee (up to 4 a day), and low-fat milk.**
- ▶ **Avoid fruit juice.**

FITNESS PROGRAM

For all strength training exercises during Week 5 to Week 8, you should aim for 3 sets of 8-12 repetitions of each exercise, using a 3 second lowering speed, 1 second pause, and a 1 second lifting speed. These are best performed with only a 60 second rest between sets.

MON

week 5
CV: 45-50mins

MON

week 6
CV: 50-55mins

TUE

CV: 20mins
ST: 3 sets of 8-12 reps

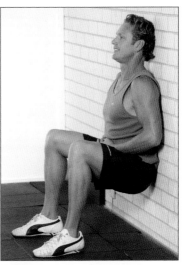

1 Ski squats

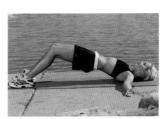

2 Hip extensions

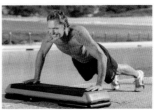

3 Hands elevated push-ups

rest day

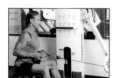

4 Seated row

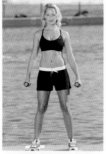

5 Lateral raise

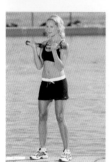

6 Dumbbell curls

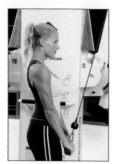

7 Tricep pushdowns

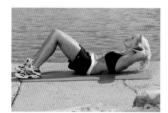

8 Sit-ups

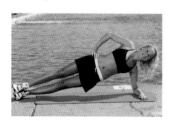

9 Side bridge

THU

week 5
CV: 40-45mins

THU

week 6
CV: 45-50mins

<table>
<tr><td>

FRI

CV: 20mins
ST: 3 sets of 8-12 reps

</td><td>

SAT

rest day

</td></tr>
</table>

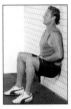
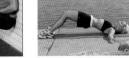

1 Ski squats   **2** Hip extensions

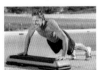

3 Hands elevated push-ups   **4** Seated row

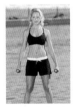
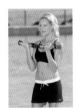
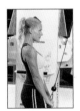

5 Lateral raise   **6** Dumbbell curls   **7** Tricep pushdowns

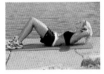
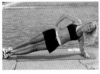

8 Sit-ups   **9** Side bridge

SUN

week 5
CV: 40mins

SUN

week 6
CV: 60mins

weeks 7 & 8

FOOD PROGRAM

WEEK 7 – CHOOSE LOW GI FOODS

Low Glycemic Index (GI) foods help control your blood sugar levels and also control your appetite so you feel fuller for longer. Recent research shows including low GI foods as part of a weight loss diet helps to maintain your metabolic rate (the speed at which you burn up kilojoules at rest) and reduces the chance of regaining weight after it has been lost.

For examples of low GI food, refer to the table on page 33.

Week 7 checklist

▸ **Switch to wholegrain bread.**

▸ **Switch to basmati or doongara rice.**

▸ **Avoid highly processed breakfast cereals. Eat porridge, natural muesli or high-fibre, wholegrain cereals.**

▸ **Choose low-fat yoghurt or fruit for snacks.**

▸ **Avoid sugary foods like lollies, cakes, biscuits, and sweets.**

▸ **If you do eat high GI foods, combine them with lower GI foods to reduce the overall GI of the meal.**

▸ **Eat sweet potato or sweet corn instead of white potatoes.**

WEEK 8 – MANAGE SPECIAL EVENTS

Social situations and special occasions can be tempting times when you are trying to lose weight. If you eat out at restaurants, there are often healthier choices on the menu. If you eat out at other people's houses, ask for smaller servings or have a light snack before you go, so you don't arrive feeling ravenous.

Week 8 checklist

▸ **Revise Week 1 to Week 7 checklists and try to maintain all your new habits.**

▸ **Choose to eat at restaurants where you know there is a variety of healthy dishes available.**

▸ **Eat something light before going out to limit overeating.**

▸ **Always order water and sip constantly throughout the meal.**

▸ **Ask for accompaniments such as plain bread, steamed rice, vegetables, or salads to fill up on.**

▸ **Ask for two entrée dishes, rather than an entrée and a main course.**

▸ **If you have dessert, choose fruit-based options.**

▸ **Minimise alcohol intake—see Week 6 to revise how to manage alcohol intake.**

▸ **If at a party, stand away from the food table.**

▸ **If eating at a buffet, use only small plates and select salads, seafood dishes, and grills.**

MON
week 7
CV: 50-55mins

TUE
CV: 25mins
ST: 3 sets of 8-12 reps

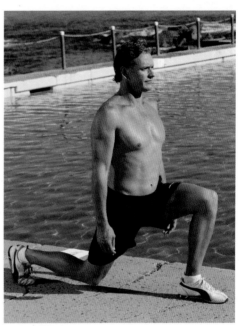

1 Static lunges

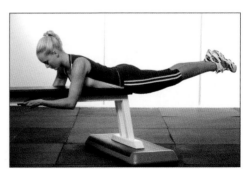

2 Reverse back extensions

MON
week 8
CV: 60mins

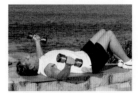

3 Dumbbell flyes

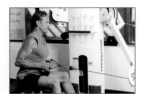

4 Seated row

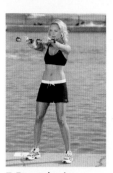

5 Frontal raise

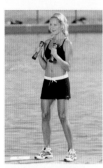

6 Hammer curls

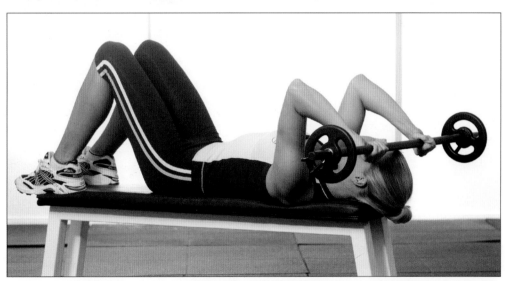

7 Lying tricep extensions

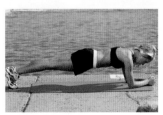

8 Front bridge

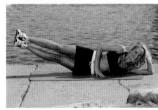

9 Side leg raise

WED

rest day

THU

week 7
CV: 45-50mins

THU

week 8
CV: 55mins

FRI

CV: 25mins
ST: 3 sets of 8-12 reps

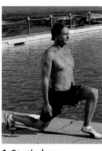

1 Static lunges

2 Reverse back extensions

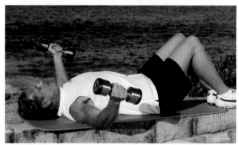

3 Dumbbell flyes

4 Seated row

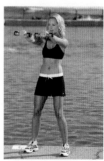

5 Frontal raise

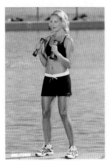

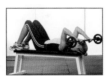

6 Hammer curls

7 Lying tricep extensions

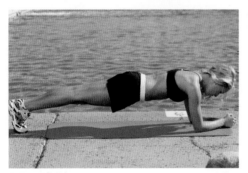

8 Front bridge

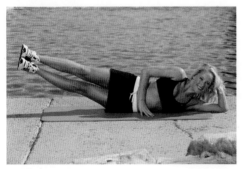

9 Side leg raise

SUN

week 7
CV: 50mins

SUN

week 8
CV: 70mins

▶ Congratulations! You have reached the end of the initial 8 weeks of your Fitsmart program and by now would have adopted new, healthy habits. Well done on all of the changes you have made—keep up the great work!

▶ If you find the rate of your weight loss has decreased, go to Plan B or C for a more structured, kilojoule-controlled approach to continue building on your weight loss results. If your weight is still reducing steadily, keep up your new habits until you reach your goal weight. At that time, you will need to start eating more of the same types of foods you are eating now, in order to maintain your weight at a new level.

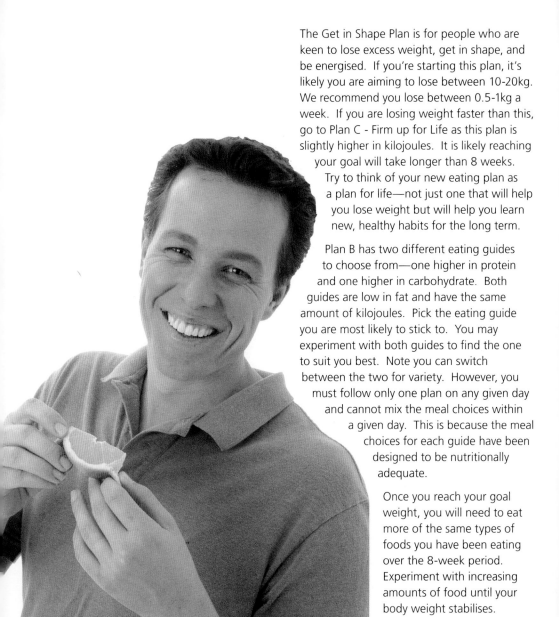

PLAN B-GET IN SHAPE

The Get in Shape Plan is for people who are keen to lose excess weight, get in shape, and be energised. If you're starting this plan, it's likely you are aiming to lose between 10-20kg. We recommend you lose between 0.5-1kg a week. If you are losing weight faster than this, go to Plan C - Firm up for Life as this plan is slightly higher in kilojoules. It is likely reaching your goal will take longer than 8 weeks. Try to think of your new eating plan as a plan for life—not just one that will help you lose weight but will help you learn new, healthy habits for the long term.

Plan B has two different eating guides to choose from—one higher in protein and one higher in carbohydrate. Both guides are low in fat and have the same amount of kilojoules. Pick the eating guide you are most likely to stick to. You may experiment with both guides to find the one to suit you best. Note you can switch between the two for variety. However, you must follow only one plan on any given day and cannot mix the meal choices within a given day. This is because the meal choices for each guide have been designed to be nutritionally adequate.

Once you reach your goal weight, you will need to eat more of the same types of foods you have been eating over the 8-week period. Experiment with increasing amounts of food until your body weight stabilises.

HIGHER CARBOHYDRATE MEAL GUIDE

▷ **Choose 1 breakfast, 1 lunch, and 1 dinner option each day plus 1 snack.**

▷ **Eat regularly. You should be eating every 3-5 hours.**

▷ **Include healthy fats in moderation. Aim for no more than 1½ tablespoons of margarine or oil per day. The margarine can be used as a spread on bread or on vegetables. The oil can be used in cooking or to make a salad dressing.**

▷ **Keep up your fluids by aiming for 2 litres (8 glasses) per day. Fluids include water, diet cordials, diet soft drinks, tea, and coffee. Water is the best choice—it contains no kilojoules, no added sugar, and no stimulants.**

▷ **Choose different meal and snack options each day. This ensures variety in your diet and keeps food interesting.**

▷ **Note: dinner meals refer to 1 serving of the recipe.**

MEAL	PLAN B (5800KJ)
Breakfast	2 slices wholegrain toast, thinly spread peanut butter + Blueberry Smoothie*
	1 cup bran cereal, 1½ tablespoons sultanas, 1 cup low-fat milk
	½ cup untoasted muesli, 200g low-fat yoghurt, 6 dried apricots
	2 wheat cereal biscuits, 1 cup low-fat milk, small banana
	1 thick slice raisin toast, thinly spread honey + 1 apple + skim milk latte
	2 slices rye toast, 2 slices low-fat cheese + 125ml fresh orange juice
	Fruity Porridge*
Lunch	1 wholemeal wrap with ½ cup chilli beans, small handful low-fat grated cheese, chopped lettuce, tomato, cucumber
	Salsa Penne*
	1 medium wholegrain roll, low-fat cottage cheese, avocado, carrot, beetroot, lettuce, gherkin
	1 vegetarian sushi hand roll + small mixed green salad, 1 tablespoon low-fat grated cheese
	1 cup basmati rice, 1 cup steamed vegetables, small handful of cashew nuts + 200g low-fat frozen yoghurt
	Winter Vegetable Soup*, mixed grain roll + 200g low-fat yoghurt
	Chickpea Salad*
Dinner	Chinese-Style Fish*
	200g grilled fish with stir-fried vegetables
	Spaghetti Bolognaise & Salad*
	Chicken Risotto*
	Veal with Pasta & Spinach*
	Jacket Potato*
	Chicken Stir-Fry*
	Oriental Salmon*
	Spicy Couscous with Lamb*
	Lamb Cutlets*
	Creamy Chicken Curry*
Snacks	1

*see recipe section

- ▸ **Choose 1 breakfast, 1 lunch, and 1 dinner option each day plus 1 snack.**
- ▸ **Eat regularly. You should be eating every 3-5 hours.**
- ▸ **Include healthy fats in moderation. Aim for no more than 1½ tablespoons of margarine or oil per day. The margarine can be used as a spread on bread or on vegetables. The oil can be used in cooking or to make a salad dressing.**
- ▸ **Keep up your fluids by aiming for 2 litres (8 glasses) per day. Fluids include water, diet cordials, diet soft drinks, tea, and coffee. Water is the best choice— it contains no kilojoules, no added sugar, and no stimulants.**
- ▸ **Choose different meal and snack options each day. This ensures you get variety in your diet and keeps food interesting.**

MEAL	PLAN B (5800 KJ)
Breakfast	2 slices multigrain toast, thinly spread jam, honey or peanut butter + 200g low-fat plain or fruit yoghurt
	1⅓ cups flaky-type cereal, 1 cup low-fat milk
	½ cup Muesli*, 3 heaped tablespoons of low-fat natural yoghurt, ½ cup low-fat milk
	1 wholegrain English muffin, thinly spread jam, honey or peanut butter + a large skim latte
	1 cup cooked porridge or rolled oats made with 1 cup low-fat milk
	1 toasted bagel, thinly spread jam, honey or peanut butter + a large skim cappuccino
	2 wheat cereal biscuits, 1 cup low-fat milk
Lunch	1 wholegrain sandwich or large grainy roll, 2 slices lean leg ham, avocado, 2 cups salad
	1 sushi hand roll with fish filling + 2 cups salad with lettuce, tomato, 1 chopped boiled egg, cucumber, carrot, capsicum, mushroom, snowpeas
	Winter Vegetable Soup* + crusty bread roll
	Chicken Salad*
	Chicken & Veg Soup* + 2 slices wholegrain bread
	Toasted bagel, 3 slices smoked salmon, rocket, thinly spread reduced-fat cream cheese, 2 cups green salad
	1 pita wrap, 2 small slices rare roast beef, thinly spread mustard, 2 cups garden salad
Dinner	Fish in Foil* + 1 cup chopped fruit salad
	Pork Stir-Fry* + 3 fresh dates
	Chicken & Veg Soup* + 1 medium pear
	Steak & Vegetables* + 1 cup sliced peaches in natural juice
	Tuna & Veg Frittata* + 1 cup chopped pineapple
	Chinese Steamed Fish* + 1 mango
	Beef & Black Bean BBQ* + 1 punnet of berries
	Lamb Salad* + 2 nectarines
	Chicken & Ginger* + 4 dried apricot halves
	Vegetable Omelette* + 1 cup diced watermelon
	Tandoori Chicken* + small handful grapes
Snacks	1

*see recipe section

weeks 1 & 2

FITNESS PROGRAM

Total days per week: 6
Cardio training days: 3
Strength training days: 3
Total time: 5-6 hours

The emphasis for this program is interval training combined with strength training. There will be 1 prolonged, easy to moderate continuous cardio session and 2 interval workouts at a higher intensity.

For all strength training exercises during Week 1 to Week 4, aim to do 2 sets of 12-15 repetitions, using a 3 second lowering speed, 2 second pause, and a 1 second lifting speed. Each set should have only 45 seconds rest in between.

The order that the strength exercises are performed is very important, so follow the same order as they are noted in the program.

For all continuous (C) cardio sessions (Sundays), training heart rates are between 70-80% of maximum (7-8 on RPE). The 2 intervals (I) sessions require the heart rate to be sustained at a higher intensity of 80-90%.

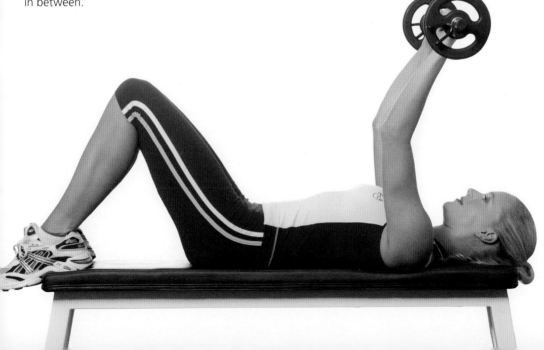

ST: 2 sets of 12-15 reps

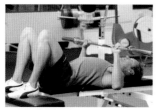

1 Bench press

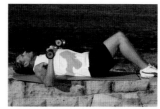

2 Dumbbell bench press

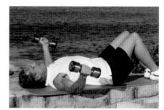

3 Dumbbell flyes

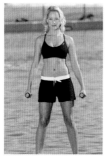

4 Lateral raise

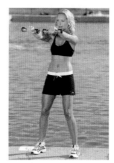

5 Frontal raise

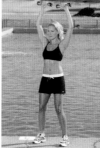

6 Dumbbell shoulder press

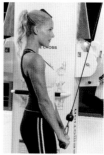

7 Tricep pushdowns

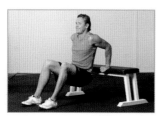

8 Dips

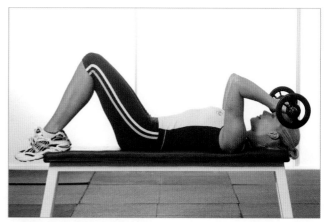

9 Lying tricep extensions

CV: 40i

Interval workouts for
Weeks 1 and 2 require
3 minutes of higher
intensity, with 3 minutes
active rest, repeated
5 times. Times include
warm-up.

ST: 2 sets of 12-15 reps

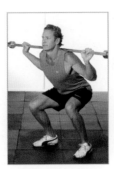

1 Barbell squats

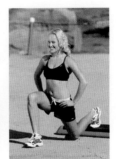

2 Bulgarian squats

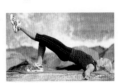

3 Single leg hip extensions

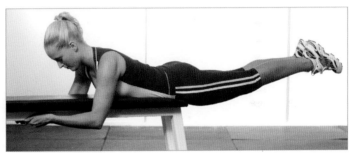

4 Reverse back extensions

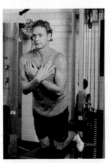

5 Modified leg curls

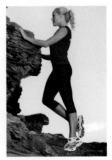

6 Single leg standing calf raise

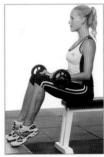

7 Bent knee calf raise

CV: 40i

ST: 2 sets of 12-15 reps

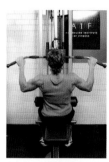

1 Lat pulldown wide grip

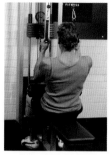

2 Lat pulldown narrow grip

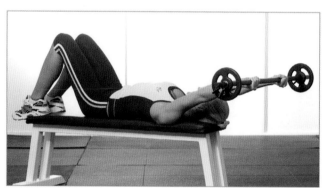

3 Barbell pullovers

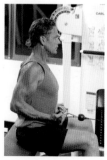

4 Seated row underhand grip

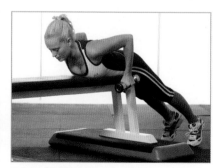

5 Dumbbell rows neutral grip

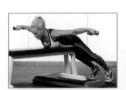

6 Prone flyes

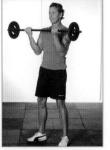

7 Barbell curls

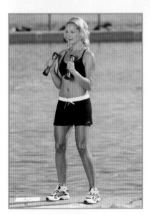

8 Hammer curls

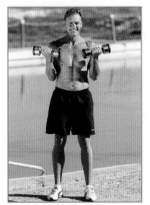

9 Dumbbell curls with a twist

rest day

SUN

week 1
CV: 50C

SUN

week 2
CV: 60C

weeks 3 & 4
ST: 2 sets of 12-15 reps

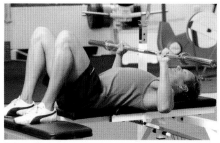

1 Bench press

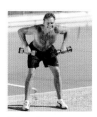

2 Bent over rows

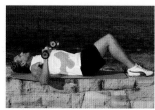

3 Dumbbell bench press

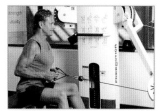

4 Seated row

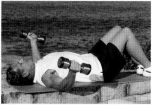

5 Dumbbell flyes

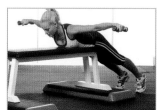

6 Prone flyes

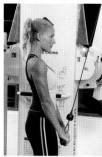

7 Tricep pushdowns

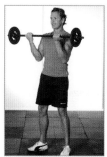

8 Barbell curls

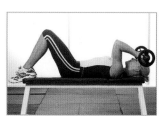

9 Lying tricep extensions

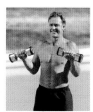

10 Reverse grip dumbbell curls

CV: 40i

Interval workouts for Weeks 3 and 4 require 5 minutes at a higher intensity, with 2 minutes active rest, repeated 5 times. Times include warm-up.

ST: 2 sets of 12-15 reps

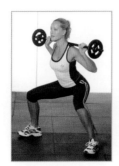
1 Wide squats

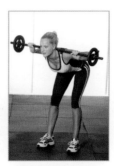
2 Good mornings

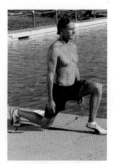
3 Dynamic lunges

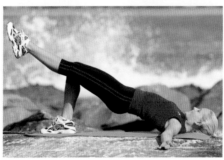
4 Single leg hip extensions

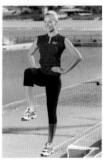
5 Step-ups

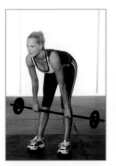
6 Romanian deadlifts

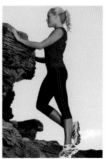
7 Single leg standing calf raise

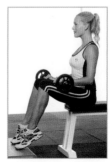
8 Bent knee calf raise

CV: 40i

ST: 2 sets of 12-15 reps

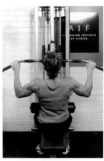

1 Lat pulldown wide grip

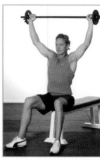

2 Barbell shoulder press

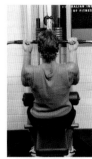

3 Lat pulldown underhand grip

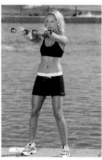

4 Frontal raise

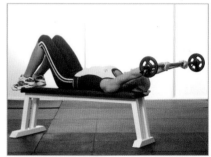

5 Barbell pullovers

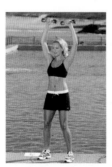

6 Dumbbell shoulder press

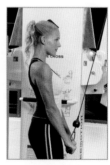

7 Tricep pushdowns

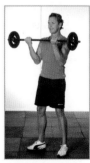

8 Barbell curls

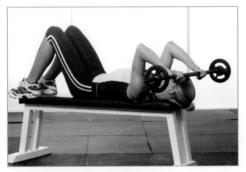
9 Lying tricep extensions

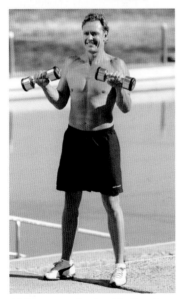
10 Reverse grip dumbbell curls

rest day

week 3
CV: 50C

week 4
CV: 70C

For all strength training exercises during Weeks 5 to 8, aim to do 3 sets of 8-10 repetitions, using a 4 second lowering speed, no pause, and a 1 second lifting speed. Each set should have 60 seconds rest in between.

ST: 3 sets of 8-10 reps

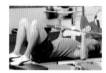

1 Bench press

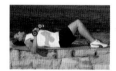

2 Dumbbell bench press

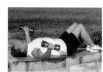

3 Dumbbell flyes

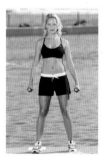

4 Lateral raise

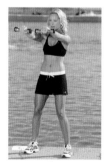

5 Frontal raise

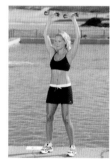

6 Dumbbell shoulder press

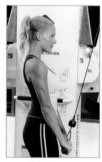

7 Tricep pushdowns

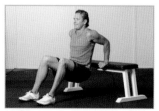

8 Dips

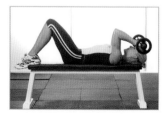

9 Lying tricep extensions

CV: 50i

ST: 3 sets of 8-10 reps

Interval workouts for
Weeks 5 and 6 require
3 minutes at a higher
intensity, with 3 minutes
active rest, repeated
6 times. Times include
warm-up.

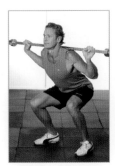

1 Barbell squats

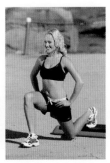

2 Bulgarian squats

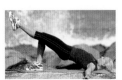

3 Single leg hip extensions

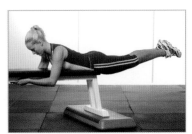

4 Reverse back extensions

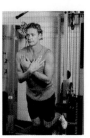

5 Modified leg curls

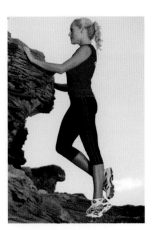

6 Single leg standing calf raise

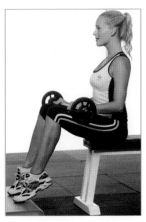

7 Bent knee calf raise

115

CV: 50i

ST: 3 sets of 8-10 reps

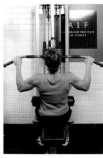

1 Lat pulldown wide grip

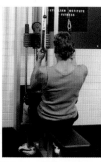

2 Lat pulldown narrow grip

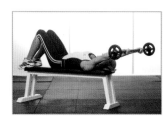

3 Barbell pullovers

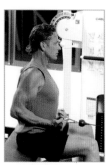

4 Seated row underhand grip

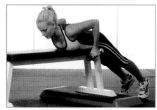

5 Dumbbell rows

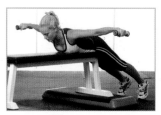

6 Prone flyes

rest day

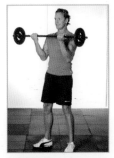

7 Barbell curls

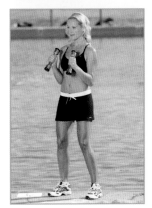

8 Hammer curls

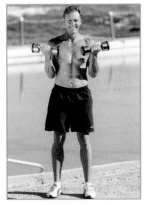

9 Dumbbell curls with a twist

week 5
CV: 60C

week 6
CV: 80C

ST: 3 sets of 8-10 reps

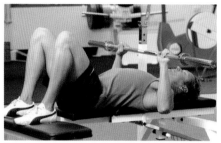

1 Bench press

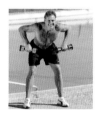

2 Bent over rows

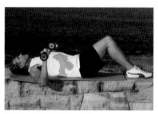

3 Dumbbell bench press

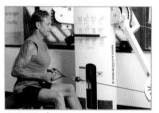

4 Seated row

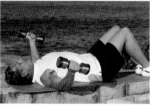

5 Dumbbell flyes

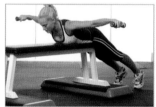

6 Prone flyes

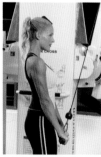

7 Tricep pushdowns

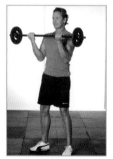

8 Barbell curls

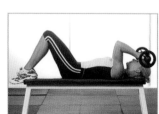

9 Lying tricep extensions

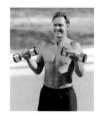

10 Reverse grip dumbbell curls

CV: 50i

Interval workouts for Weeks 7 and 8 require 5 minutes at a higher intensity, with 2 minutes active rest, repeated 6 times. Times include warm-up.

ST: 3 sets of 8-10 reps

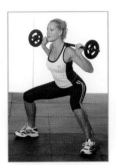

1 Wide squats

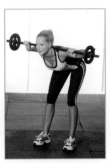

2 Good mornings

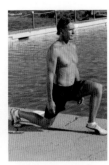

3 Dynamic lunges

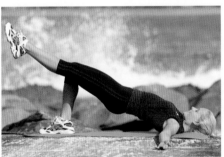

4 Single leg hip extensions

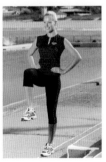

5 Step-ups

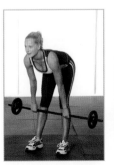

6 Romanian deadlifts

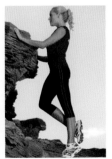

7 Single leg standing calf raise

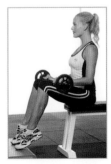

8 Bent knee calf raise

CV: 50i

ST: 3 sets of 8-10 reps

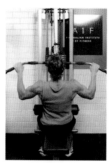

1 Lat pulldown wide grip

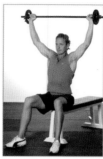

2 Barbell shoulder press

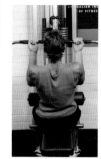

3 Lat pulldown underhand grip

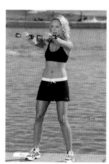

4 Frontal raise

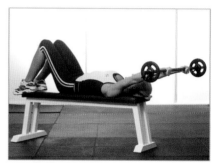

5 Barbell pullovers

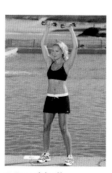

6 Dumbbell shoulder press

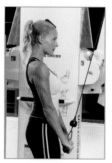

7 Tricep pushdowns

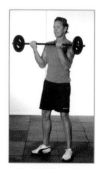

8 Barbell curls

rest day

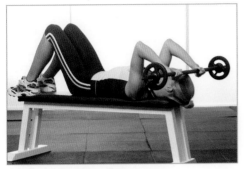

9 Lying tricep extensions

week 7
CV: 70C

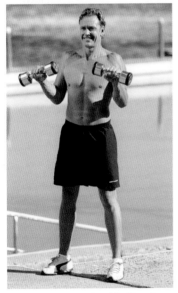

10 Reverse grip dumbbell curls

week 8
CV: 90C

The Firm up for Life Plan is for people who are already active, but want to tone up and look trim. If you're starting this plan it's likely you are aiming to lose 5-10kg. By achieving this, you will reduce your body fat level enough to feel toned and trim. While different people lose weight at different rates, we recommend you lose around 0.5kg a week on this plan. A slower rate of weight loss on this plan is recommended to ensure the weight you lose is body fat and not muscle. You'll also need to ensure you have enough energy to keep up your activity level. If you find you are losing weight faster than this, add in an extra snack during the day and monitor your progress.

Within the Firm up for Life Plan, you have 2 different eating guides to choose from— 1 higher in protein and 1 higher in carbohydrate. Both are low in fat and have the same amount of kilojoules. Pick the eating guide you are most likely to stick to. Experiment with both guides to find the one that suits you best. Note you can switch between the two, however you must be following only one guide on any given day and cannot mix the meal choices within a given day. This is because the meal choices for each plan have been designed so that in combination, they are nutritionally adequate.

Once you reach your goal weight, you will need to eat more of the same types of foods you have been eating over the 8-week period. Experiment with increasing amounts of food until your body weight stabilises.

HIGHER CARBOHYDRATE MEAL GUIDE

▸ **Choose 1 breakfast, 1 lunch, and 1 dinner option each day plus 2 snacks.**

▸ **Eat regularly. You should be eating every 3-5 hours.**

▸ **Include healthy fats in moderation. Aim for no more than 1½ tablespoons of margarine or oil per day. The margarine can be used as a spread on bread or on vegetables. The oil can be used in cooking or to make a salad dressing.**

▸ **Keep up your fluids by aiming for 2 litres (8 glasses) per day. Fluids include water, diet cordials, diet soft drinks, tea, and coffee. Water is the best choice—it contains no kilojoules, no added sugar, and no stimulants.**

▸ **Choose different meal and snack options each day. This ensures variety in your diet and keeps food interesting.**

MEAL	PLAN C (7,650KJ)
Breakfast	2 slices wholegrain toast, thinly spread peanut butter + Blueberry Smoothie*
	1⅓ cups bran cereal, 1½ tablespoons sultanas, 1 cup low-fat milk
	½ cup untoasted muesli, 200g low-fat yoghurt, 6 dried apricots
	2 wheat cereal biscuits, 1 cup low-fat milk, 1 small banana
	1 thick slice raisin toast, thinly spread honey + 1 apple + a skinny latte
	2 slices rye toast, 2 slices low-fat cheese + 125ml fresh orange juice
	Fruity Porridge*
Lunch	1 wholemeal wrap, ½ cup chilli beans, small handful low-fat grated cheese, chopped lettuce, tomato, cucumber + small glass of fresh strawberry juice
	1 vegetarian sushi hand roll + small mixed green salad, small handful low-fat grated cheese + ½ cup rice salad + 1 mandarin
	1 medium wholegrain roll, low-fat cottage cheese, avocado, carrot, beetroot, lettuce, gherkin + 1 larger wholegrain roll + small banana
	Salsa Penne* + 1 cup raspberries
	1½ cups basmati rice, 1 cup steamed vegetables, small handful cashew nuts + 200g low-fat frozen yoghurt + small tub of fruit in natural juice
	Winter Vegetable Soup* with mixed grain roll + 200g low-fat yoghurt + 1 pear
	Chickpea Salad* + small handful grapes
Dinner	200g grilled fish with stir-fried vegetables
	Chinese-Style Fish* + 2 guavas or other small fruit
	Spaghetti Bolognaise & Salad* + 1 cup mixed berries
	Chicken Risotto* + 1 grapefruit
	Veal with Pasta & Spinach* + 1 orange
	Jacket Potato* + 1 persimmon or kiwi fruit
	Chicken Stir-Fry* + 2 apricots
	Oriental Salmon* + 1 cup raspberries
	Spicy Couscous with Lamb* + 1 small banana
	Lamb Cutlets* + 1 cup watermelon
	Creamy Chicken Curry* + 1½ tablespoons sultanas
Snacks	2

*see recipe section

HIGHER PROTEIN MEAL GUIDE

▶ **Choose 1 breakfast, 1 lunch, and 1 dinner option each day plus 2 snacks.**

▶ **Eat regularly. You should be eating every 3-5 hours.**

▶ **Include healthy fats in moderation. Aim for no more than 1½ tablespoons of margarine or oil per day. The margarine can be used as a spread on bread or on vegetables. The oil can be used in cooking or to make a salad dressing.**

▶ **Keep up your fluids by aiming for 2 litres (8 glasses) per day. Fluids include water, diet cordials, diet soft drinks, tea and coffee. Water is the best choice—it contains no kilojoules, no added sugar, and no stimulants.**

▶ **Choose different meal and snack options each day. This ensures variety in your diet and keeps food interesting.**

▶ **Note: dinner meals refer to 1 serving from recipe.**

MEAL	PLAN C (7650 KJ)
Breakfast	2 slices multigrain toast, thinly spread jam, honey or peanut butter, 200g low-fat plain or fruit yoghurt + 1 medium apple, pear, banana, or orange
	1⅓ cups flaky-type cereal, 1 cup low-fat milk, 1 cup chopped pineapple, melon, or fruit salad
	½ cup Muesli*, 3 heaped tablespoons low-fat natural yoghurt, ½ cup low-fat milk + 3 prunes or dates or 1½ tablespoons sultanas
	1 wholegrain English muffin, thinly spread jam, honey or peanut butter + small low-fat fruit smoothie
	1 cup of cooked porridge or rolled oats made with 1 cup low-fat milk + 1½ tablespoons sultanas, currants, or raisins
	1 Blueberry Bagel*
	2 wheat cereal biscuits, 1 cup low-fat milk + 1 cup peach or apricot slices in natural juice
Lunch	1 wholegrain sandwich or large grainy roll, 3 slices lean leg ham, 1 tablespoon avocado, 2 cups garden salad + 200g low-fat yoghurt
	1 sushi hand roll with fish filling + 2 cups salad with lettuce, tomato, 2 chopped boiled eggs, cucumber, carrot, capsicum, mushroom, snowpeas + ½ handful grated low-fat cheese
	1½ cups Winter Vegetable Soup* + 1 crusty bread roll + large skim cappuccino
	Chicken Salad*
	Chicken & Veg Soup*, 1 cup stir-fried vegetables + 200g frozen low-fat yoghurt
	Toasted bagel, 4 slices smoked salmon, rocket, thinly spread low-fat cream cheese, 2 cups green salad + a large skim latte
	1 pita wrap, 3 small slices rare roast beef, thinly spread mustard, 2 cups garden salad + 200g low-fat yoghurt
Dinner	Fish in Foil* + 1 cup chopped fruit salad
	Pork Stir-Fry* + 3 fresh dates or prunes
	Chicken & Veg Soup* + 1 medium pear or apple
	Steak & Vegetables* + 1 cup sliced peaches in natural juice
	Tuna & Veg Frittata* + 1 cup chopped pineapple or melon
	Chinese Steamed Fish* + 1 mango or orange
	Beef & Black Bean BBQ* + 1 punnet of berries
	Lamb Salad* + 2 nectarines or kiwi fruit
	Chicken & Ginger* + 4 dried apricot halves or 3 dried apple rings
	Vegetable Omelette* + 1 cup diced watermelon or rockmelon
	Tandoori Chicken* + small handful grapes
Snacks	2

*see recipe

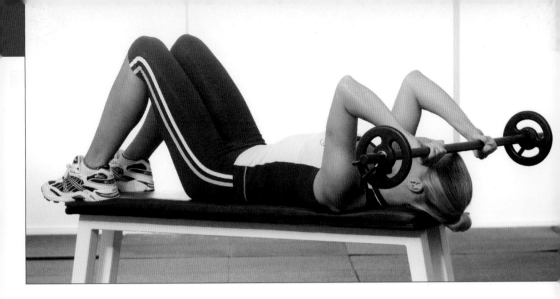

weeks 1 & 2

FITNESS PROGRAM

Total days per week: 6
Cardio training days: 4
Strength/cardio training days: 2
Total time: 5-6 hours

The emphasis for this program is a combination of strength training and cardiovascular training; continuous cardio work; multi-mode cardio work, and interval training. The cardio component focuses on having 2 prolonged, easy-to-moderate, continuous sessions and 2 interval workouts at a higher intensity.

For all strength exercises during Week 1 to Week 4, aim to do 3 sets of 15-20 repetitions, using a 2 second lowering speed, 1 second pause, and a 1 second lifting speed. Each set should have a 45 second rest in between.

The order that the strength exercises are performed is very important, so follow the same order as they are noted in the program.

To increase energy expenditure, strength will be interspersed with short bursts of cardio.

For all continuous cardio sessions (Wednesdays and Sundays), training heart rates are between 70-80% of maximum (or 7-8 on RPE). The 2 intervals sessions require the heart rate to be sustained at 85-95% of maximum.

ST: 3 sets of 15-20 reps

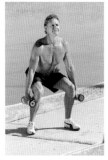

1 Dumbbell squats

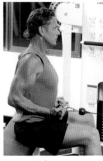

2 Seated row underhand grip

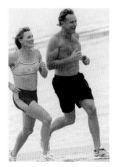

3 Cardio

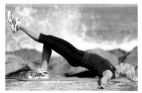

4 Single leg hip extensions

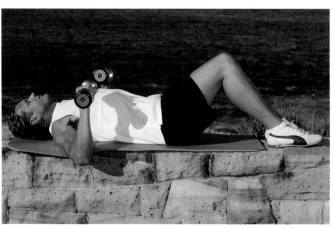

5 Dumbbell bench press

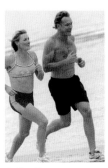

6 Cardio

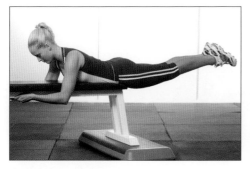

7 Reverse back extensions

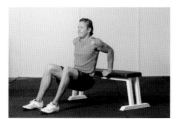

8 Dips

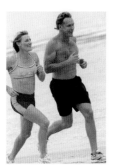

9 Cardio

TUE

CV: 40i

Interval workouts for Weeks 1 and 2 require 4 minutes at a higher intensity, with 1 minute active rest, repeated 6 times. Times include warm-up.

WED

week 1
CV: 40C

WED

week 2
CV: 40C

ST: 3 sets of 15-20 reps

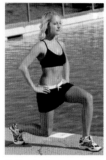

1 Static lunges

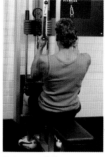

2 Lat pulldown narrow grip

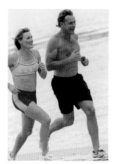

3 Cardio

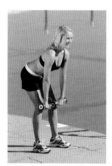

4 Dumbbell Romanian deadlifts

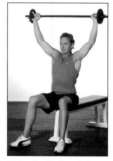

5 Barbell shoulder press

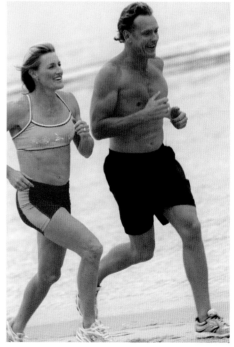

6 Cardio

CV: 45i

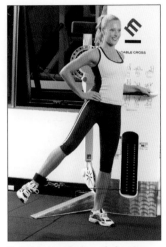

7 Cable single leg abductions

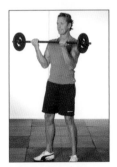

8 Barbell curls

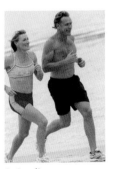

9 Cardio

SAT

rest day

SUN

week 1
CV: 60C

SUN

week 2
CV: 70C

MON
weeks 3 & 4
ST: 3 sets of 15-20 reps

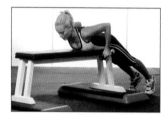

1 Dumbbell rows

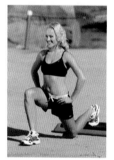

2 Bulgarian squats

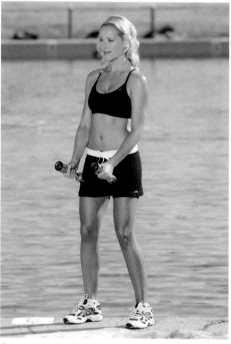

3 Hammer curls

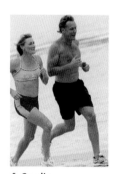

4 Cardio

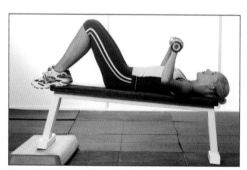

5 Decline dumbbell press

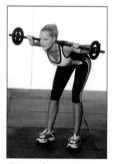

6 Good mornings

CV: 40i

Interval workouts for Weeks 3 and 4 require 1 minute at a higher intensity, with 4 minutes active rest, repeated 6 times. Times include warm-up.

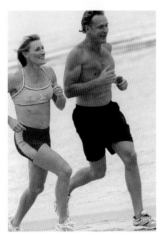

7 Overhead tricep extensions

WED
week 3
CV: 45C

8 Cardio

WED
week 4
CV: 50C

ST: 3 sets of 15-20 reps

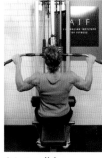

1 Lat pulldown wide grip

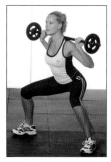

2 Wide squats

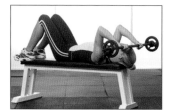

3 Lying tricep extensions

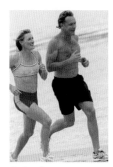

4 Cardio

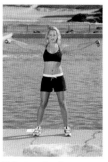

5 Lateral raise

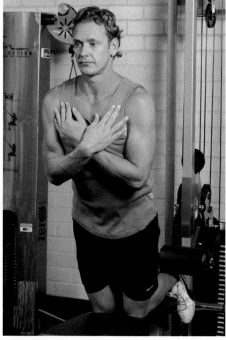

6 Modified leg curls

CV: 40i

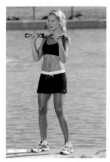

7 Zottman curls

SAT

rest day

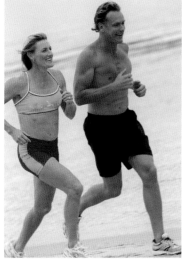

8 Cardio

SUN

week 3
CV: 60C

SUN

week 4
CV: 80C

MON
weeks 5 & 6

For all strength training (ST) exercises during Weeks 5 to 8, aim to do 4 sets of 10-12 repetitions, using a 3 second lowering speed, 2 second pause and a 2 second lifting speed. Each set should have a 30 second rest in between.

Intersperse ST exercises with 60 seconds of high intensity of CV exercise.

ST: 4 sets of 10-12 reps

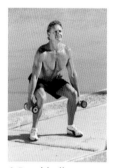

1 Dumbbell squats

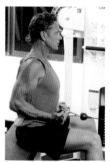

2 Seated row underhand grip

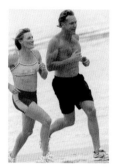

3 Cardio

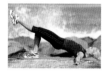

4 Single leg hip extensions

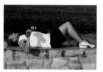

5 Dumbbell bench press

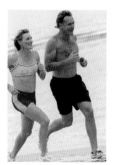

6 Cardio

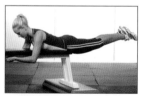

7 Reverse back extensions

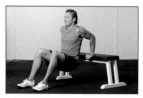

8 Dips

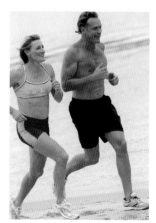

9 Cardio

TUE

CV: 40i

Interval workouts for Weeks 5 and 6 require 4 minutes at a higher intensity, with 1 minute active rest, repeated 7 times. Times include warm-up.

WED

week 5
CV: 50C

WED

week 6
CV: 55C

THU

ST: 4 sets of 10-12 reps

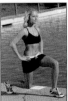 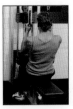 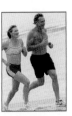

1 Static lunges **2** Lat pulldown narrow grip **3** Cardio

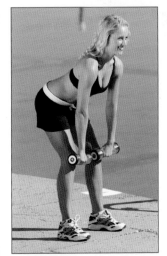 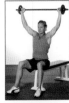

5 Barbell shoulder press

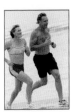

4 Dumbbell Romanian deadlifts **6** Cardio

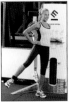 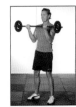 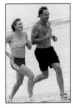

7 Cable single leg abductions **8** Barbell curls **9** Cardio

135

FRI

CV: 40i

SAT

rest day

SUN

week 5
CV: 70C

SUN

week 6
CV: 90C

MON

weeks 7 & 8
ST: 4 sets of 10-12 reps

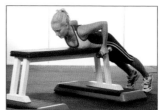

1 Dumbbell rows

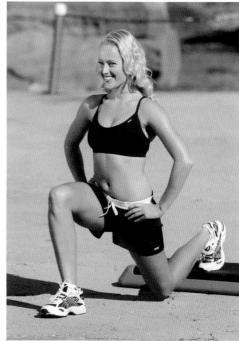

2 Bulgarian squats

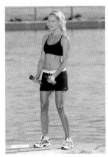

3 Hammer curls

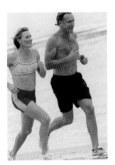

4 Cardio

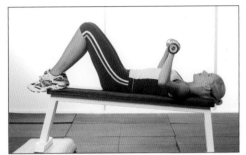

5 Decline dumbbell press

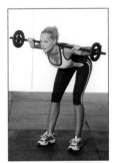

6 Good mornings

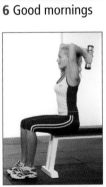

7 Overhead tricep
extensions

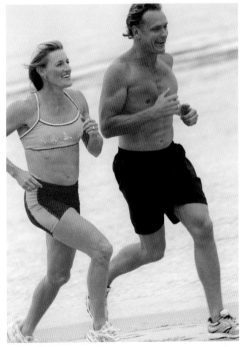

8 Cardio

TUE

CV: 40i

Interval workouts for Week 7 and Week 8 require 1 minute at a higher intensity, with 4 minutes active rest, repeated 7 times.

WED

week 7

CV: 55C

WED

week 8

CV: 60C

THU

ST: 4 sets of 10-12 reps

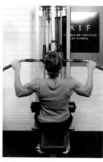 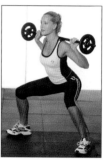

1 Lat pulldown wide grip   **2** Wide squats

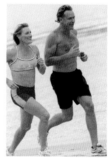 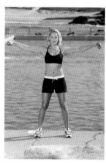

4 Cardio   **5** Lateral raise

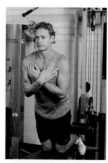 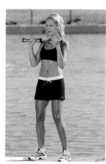

6 Modified leg curls   **7** Zottman curls

CV: 40i

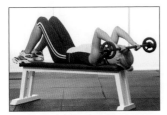

3 Lying tricep extensions

rest day

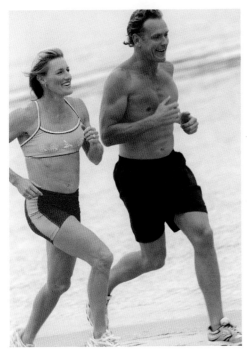

8 Cardio

week 7
CV: 80C

week 8
CV: 100C

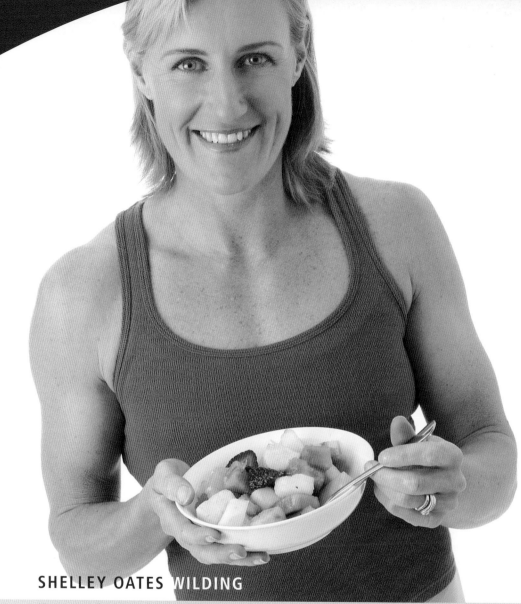

SHELLEY OATES WILDING

'Every Sunday night I sit down, I have a diary, and I make sure that I have all the things in there that are important to me. So the first thing is obviously my family and then my training is all booked in before I fill up my free time.'

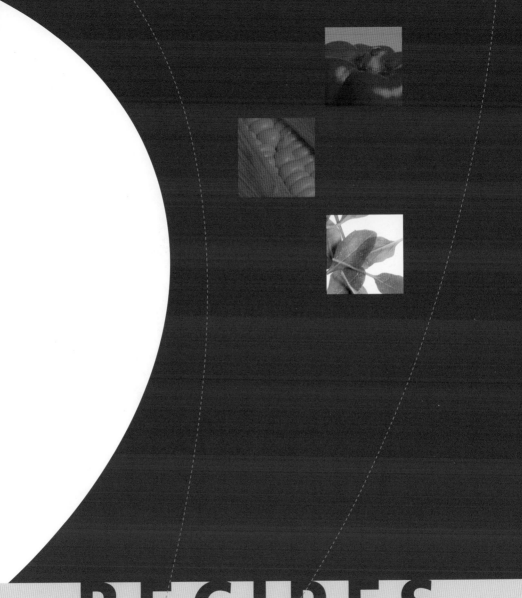

RECIPES

breakfast

HIGHER CARBOHYDRATE PLAN B

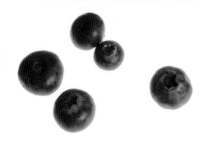

Blueberry Smoothie

Serves 2

1 cup blueberries* (fresh or frozen)
1 tbsp wheatgerm
2 tsp honey
1 cup low-fat soy milk (or skim if preferred)

Place all ingredients in a blender and blend for 1 minute until smooth. Pour into a glass and serve immediately.

Plan C – as above

Nutritional analysis per serve	PLAN B & C
Energy (kJ)	875
Protein (g)	9
Fat (g)	1.4
Carbohydrate (g)	41
Fibre (g)	5
Sodium (mg)	195

* Other berries can be substituted for blueberries

Fruity Porridge

Serves 1

½ cup uncooked rolled oats
1 cup low-fat milk
1 tbsp sultanas
3 tbsp canned pie apples
½ tsp cinnamon
¼ tsp ground cloves

Place all ingredients in a microwave-proof bowl. Heat for approximately 2 minutes on high. Stop once to stir.

Plan C – as above

Nutritional analysis per serve	PLAN B & C
Energy (kJ)	1456
Protein (g)	15
Fat (g)	7
Carbohydrate (g)	56
Fibre (g)	4
Sodium (mg)	132

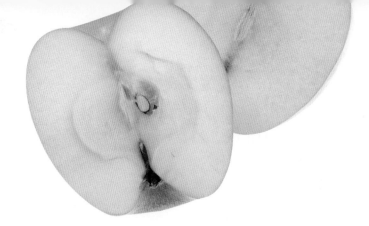

Muesli

Serves 32

8 cups rolled oats
2 cups extruded bran cereal or bran sticks
300g slivered almonds
1 cup raw pepitas (or pumpkin seeds)
1 cup raw sunflower seeds, hulled
1 cup dried apricots, roughly chopped
½ cup raisins, roughly chopped
½ cup dried currants
1 cup skim or low-fat milk per serve

Combine all ingredients except milk in an airtight container. Shake well until combined. Serve with ice-cold milk.

Plan C variation

+ 1 cup peach slices, in natural juice, per serve

Serve topped with peaches.

Nutritional analysis per serve	PLAN B	PLAN C
Energy (kJ)	1327	1687
Protein (g)	17	19
Fat (g)	12	12
Carbohydrate (g)	36	55
Fibre (g)	5	8
Sodium (mg)	136	147

Blueberry Bagel

Serves 1

1 blueberry bagel
¼ cup low-fat natural or vanilla flavoured yoghurt
¼ cup low-fat ricotta cheese
¼ tsp cinnamon

Slice bagel in half lengthways and toast cut side until golden. Mix yoghurt and ricotta until smooth. Spread toasted bagel thickly with ricotta/yoghurt mixture and sprinkle with cinnamon.

Plan C variation

+ 2 fresh dates, finely chopped.

Add dates to ricotta and yoghurt mixture.

Nutritional analysis per serve	PLAN B	PLAN C
Energy (kJ)	1543	1745
Protein (g)	20	21
Fat (g)	7	7
Carbohydrate (g)	55	67
Fibre (g)	3	5
Sodium (mg)	618	621

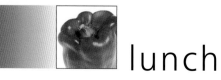

lunch

HIGHER CARBOHYDRATE PLAN B

Salsa Penne

Serves 4

2 cups pasta, uncooked
1 large onion, chopped
2 cloves garlic, chopped
2 tbsp olive oil
500g tinned tomatoes, chopped
1 cup fresh basil leaves
1 cup parmesan cheese, grated
black pepper to taste

**Cook pasta according to instructions.
Fry onion and garlic in olive oil until softened.
Add tomatoes and basil, and heat through.
Mix pasta with tomato mixture and top with
parmesan cheese and black pepper.**

Plan C variation
3½ cups pasta, uncooked

Note: *This recipe can be made in advance
and frozen in individual lunch portions.*

Nutritional analysis per serve	PLAN B	PLAN C
Energy (kJ)	1787	2152
Protein (g)	18	21
Fat (g)	17	17
Carbohydrate (g)	51	69
Fibre (g)	6	7
Sodium (mg)	426	468

Chickpea Salad

Serves 1

2 tsp water
2 small onions
1 clove garlic
1 cup canned chickpeas, drained
1 small tomato
1 tbsp tomato paste
1 dried date
3 tbsp water
½ tbsp fresh mint
1 tbsp coriander
3 cups raw spinach
2½ tbsp feta, reduced fat
10 raw almonds, chopped

**Combine water, onion, and garlic in large
pan. Cook until onion is soft. Stir in chickpeas,
tomato paste, and date, then extra water, and
herbs. Simmer with lid for 10 minutes. Stir
in spinach, simmer, uncovered, for 5 minutes
until spinach is just wilted.
Add feta and almonds.**

Plan C variation
1½ cups canned chickpeas, drained

Nutritional analysis per serve	PLAN B	PLAN C
Energy (kJ)	1789	2141
Protein (g)	32	37
Fat (g)	17	19
Carbohydrate (g)	37	48
Fibre (g)	16	21
Sodium (mg)	1185	1402

HIGHER PROTEIN PLAN B

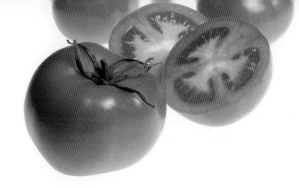

Winter Vegetable Soup

Serves 4

2 tbsp olive oil
3 onions, finely diced
3 cloves garlic, crushed
2 zucchinis, diced
4 celery stalks, sliced
2 carrots, diced
4 cups chicken stock, salt-reduced
2 cups 3-bean mix or chickpeas

**Heat oil in a large saucepan, and cook garlic
and onion until softened. Add vegetables
and stir. Add stock and bring to boil. Simmer
until vegetables are very soft. Add beans and
heat through. Serve with a crusty bread roll.**

Plan C variation

8 cups chicken stock, salt-reduced
3 cups 3-bean mix or chickpeas, or 2 cups soup
   mix or split peas
+ 4 potatoes, peeled and diced

Note: *This recipe can be made in advance
and frozen in individual lunch portions.*

Nutritional analysis per serve*	PLAN B*	PLAN C*
Energy (kJ)	1396	2000
Protein (g)	12	18
Fat (g)	13	17
Carbohydrate (g)	42	64
Fibre (g)	10	14
Sodium (mg)	1454	1581

*includes 1 bread roll

Chicken Salad

Serves 1

85g skinless cooked chicken, cut into strips
1 cup torn mixed lettuce leaves
½ cup mixed green vegetables
   (sliced cucumber, snowpeas, alfalfa sprouts)
½ cup other mixed vegetables
   (chopped tomato, carrot, capsicum, mushroom)
½ cup corn kernels or 3-bean mix
½ tbsp olive oil
½ tbsp balsamic vinegar

**Combine leaves, vegetables, and corn or beans
in a bowl. Drizzle with olive oil, sprinkle with
vinegar and serve with chicken.**

Plan C variation

Chicken & Greek Salad

+ 60g reduced-fat feta cheese, cut into cubes
   or crumbled. Mix through salad. Swap olive
   oil for 6 whole olives.

Nutritional analysis per serve	PLAN B	PLAN C
Energy (kJ)	1686	2271
Protein (g)	34	50
Fat (g)	17	26
Carbohydrate (g)	27	27
Fibre (g)	10	10
Sodium (mg)	496	1156

dinner

HIGHER CARBOHYDRATE PLAN B

Chicken Risotto

Serves 2

1 tbsp oil
200g chicken breast, diced
1 cup mushrooms, sliced
2 spring onions, sliced
⅔ cup risotto rice, uncooked
2 cups chicken stock
1 cup water
2 tbsp parmesan cheese, grated
4 cups mixed green salad

Heat half the oil in a large saucepan and stir-fry chicken until cooked. Add mushrooms and spring onions and cook for 1-2 minutes, then remove. Add remaining oil and stir-fry rice for 3 minutes. Add 1 cup stock and stir until liquid is absorbed. Continue this process until all liquid is used. Add chicken mixture and stir. Stir through cheese, and serve with green salad.

Plan C variation
400g chicken breast, diced

Nutritional analysis per serve	PLAN B	PLAN C
Energy (kJ)	2350	2917
Protein (g)	34	56
Fat (g)	24	29
Carbohydrate (g)	53	53
Fibre (g)	8	8
Sodium (mg)	806	865

Chinese-Style Fish

Serves 2

1 tbsp sesame oil
1 tbsp soy sauce
1 tsp garlic, crushed
1 tsp sugar
1 tsp ginger, grated
2½ cups cooked Jasmine rice
200g ocean perch
3 cups bok choy
2½ cups snowpeas
1 medium spring onion, sliced
1 tsp sesame seeds

Combine sesame oil, soy sauce, garlic, sugar, and ginger. Cook rice and keep warm. Place fish in steamer insert. Pour over half the dressing. Steam for about 8 minutes. Steam vegetables towards the last 4 minutes.

To serve: Spoon rice onto plate, place fish on top, and arrange vegetables. Pour over remaining dressing. Sprinkle with shallots and sesame seeds.

Plan C variation
400g ocean perch

Nutritional analysis per serve	PLAN B	PLAN C
Energy (kJ)	2278	2842
Protein (g)	29	47
Fat (g)	12	12
Carbohydrate (g)	81	94
Fibre (g)	6	7
Sodium (mg)	776	909

Spaghetti Bolognaise

Serves 2

½ brown onion
1 clove garlic, crushed
½ small carrot, finely chopped
½ celery stalk, finely chopped
200g lean minced beef
1 cup (250ml) bottled tomato pasta sauce
¼ cup (65ml) beef stock
150g uncooked spaghetti (3 cups cooked)

Mixed Spinach Salad

2 cups spinach leaves
1 medium yellow capsicum, chopped
1 small onion, sliced
balsamic vinegar to taste
½ tsp dried oregano

Cook onion and garlic in a heated non-stick
frying pan, stirring until softened. Add carrot
and celery. Cook, stirring, until tender. Add
beef, stir until changed in colour. Add sauce
and stock, and boil. Simmer uncovered for
5 minutes or until the mixture thickens.
Cook spaghetti. Combine salad ingredients
and set aside.

To serve: Pile spaghetti in shallow bowls and
top with sauce. Serve salad on small side plates.

Plan C variation

400g lean minced beef

Nutritional analysis per serve	PLAN B	PLAN C
Energy (kJ)	2418	3018
Protein (g)	37	57
Fat (g)	15	22
Carbohydrate (g)	73	73
Fibre (g)	9	9
Sodium (mg)	716	779

Veal with Pasta & Spinach

Serves 2

1 cup English spinach
1 medium brown onion, finely chopped
4 cloves garlic, finely chopped
1 tbsp olive oil
3 tbsp reduced-fat plain yoghurt
¼ tsp pepper
2 tbsp reduced-fat feta cheese
2½ cups angel hair pasta, uncooked
200g veal leg steak
4 (160g) yellow squash
⅔ cup sweet potato

Wash spinach, place in an air-tight container
with some water, and steam until limp.
Squeeze out excess liquid and chop finely.
Sauté onion and garlic in half the oil until soft.
Add spinach, yoghurt, pepper, then crumble
in feta. Cook pasta, and stir through. Pan-
fry veal in a non-stick pan with remaining oil,
about 3 minutes. Halve squash. Peel sweet
potato, and cut into 1cm wedges. Steam until
just cooked.

To serve: Pile pasta into shallow bowls with
the veal to one side. Serve vegetables in
a separate bowl.

Plan C variation

400g veal leg steak

Nutritional analysis per serve	PLAN B	PLAN C
Energy (kJ)	2340	2907
Protein (g)	39	66
Fat (g)	16	19
Carbohydrate (g)	63	63
Fibre (g)	13	13
Sodium (mg)	379	487

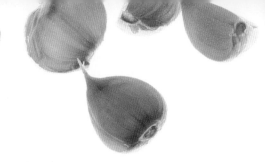

Jacket Potato

Serves 2

2 medium potatoes, unpeeled
3 cups lettuce, torn
1 small Lebanese cucumber, chopped
20 cherry tomatoes, halved
2 tbsp salad dressing
210g tuna in spring water
210g corn kernels
125g canned or fresh capsicum
2 spring onions, chopped
4 tbsp low-fat mayonnaise

**Microwave whole potatoes on high for
10 minutes. Leave to stand. Combine lettuce,
cucumber, and tomatoes. Toss dressing through
and serve on plates. Combine drained tuna,
corn, capsicum, onions (save some for garnish),
and mayonnaise. Season with pepper. Place
potato on salad and cut open. Spoon over
topping and garnish with spring onion.**

Plan C variation
510g tuna in spring water

Nutritional analysis per serve	PLAN B	PLAN C
Energy (kJ)	2264	3041
Protein (g)	36	74
Fat (g)	19	23
Carbohydrate (g)	55	55
Fibre (g)	13	13
Sodium (mg)	740	863

Chicken Stir-Fry

Serves 2

200g chicken breast, thinly sliced
1 tbsp olive oil
1 small red onion, quartered
4½ cups bok choy, halved lengthways
1¼ cups green beans, cut into thirds
2 cups fresh asparagus, halved
1 tbsp black bean sauce
½ cup water
2 tsp honey
2 tbsp soy sauce
1 tsp fresh grated ginger
2 tsp cornflour
3 cups cooked wild rice

**Cook chicken until browned and cooked
through, then remove from heat. Heat oil
in same pan and cook onion until soft. Add
vegetables and cook until tender. Combine
next 6 ingredients, and stir through. Return
chicken to pan. Stir over heat until mixture
thickens. Serve with wild rice.**

Plan C variation
450g chicken breast, thinly sliced

Nutritional analysis per serve	PLAN B	PLAN C
Energy (kJ)	2242	2963
Protein (g)	39	66
Fat (g)	16	23
Carbohydrate (g)	58	58
Fibre (g)	11	11g
Sodium (mg)	1258	1331

Oriental Salmon

Serves 2

2 x 100g salmon fillets
½ tbsp sesame oil
2 tsp fresh ginger, grated
zest of half a lemon
⅛ tsp freshly ground pepper
2 tsp nigella or sesame seeds
½ medium onion, thinly sliced
3 cups mixed, vegetables thinly sliced
1 clove garlic, crushed
2 tsp Thai fish sauce
juice of half a lemon
2 cups fresh Hokkien noodles

Sprinkle salmon (skin side down) with half sesame oil, half ginger, half lemon zest, and pepper, and leave to marinate. Heat seeds in a dry non-stick pan until roasted and aromatic, and set aside. Heat remaining oil in a non-stick pan. Stir-fry onion, then add vegetables. Add garlic, fish sauce, lemon juice, remaining zest, and ginger. Add noodles and stir. Reduce heat to very low. Heat a non-stick pan, spray with oil, and cook salmon. Place noodles on plates, lay salmon on the top, and garnish with nigella seeds.

Plan C variation
2 x 225g salmon fillets

Nutritional analysis per serve	PLAN B	PLAN C
Energy (kJ)	2220	2963
Protein (g)	30	55
Fat (g)	24	33
Carbohydrate (g)	47	47
Fibre (g)	10	10
Sodium (mg)	1381	1436

Spicy Couscous with Lamb

Serves 2

1 tbsp olive oil
1 medium onion, diced
1 clove garlic, finely chopped
1 red capsicum, chopped
1 medium zucchini, chopped
1 celery stalk, diced
1 cup red cabbage, chopped
½ medium carrot, chopped
1 tsp ground coriander
1 tsp ground cumin
1 tsp sweet paprika
2¾ cups boiling water
2 stock cubes (beef or chicken)
2 x 100g lean lamb steaks
1 sprig fresh coriander

Heat half the oil in a large saucepan. Add onions and cook until softened. Add vegetables, garlic and spices, and cook for 5 minutes, stirring. Dissolve stock cubes in water. Add 1¾ cups stock and boil. Reduce heat and cover. Cook until vegetables are tender. Heat a non-stick pan and cook lamb steaks, turning occasionally (around 10 minutes). Place couscous in a bowl. Pour over remaining oil and stock. Cover and set aside for 5 minutes until water is absorbed. Use a fork to separate. Serve couscous in bowls. Spoon sauce over. Slice steaks into strips and place on the top. Garnish with coriander.

Plan C variation
2 x 200g lean lamb steaks

Nutritional analysis per serve	PLAN B	PLAN C
Energy (kJ)	2388	3134
Protein (g)	41	70
Fat (g)	17	24
Carbohydrate (g)	62	62
Fibre (g)	690	756
Sodium (mg)	6	6

Lamb Cutlets

Serves 2

6 x 30g lamb cutlets, trimmed of fat
2 cloves garlic, crushed
2 sprigs fresh rosemary
1 tbsp olive oil
salt and pepper to taste

Sweet Potato Mash
1 large sweet potato, peeled, cubed
1 clove garlic, crushed
1 tsp dried oregano
2 tbsp low-fat or skim milk

Corn Salad
210g canned corn, drained and rinsed
3 cups mixed greens
100g cherry tomatoes, halved
balsamic vinegar

Tenderise lamb to desired thickness. Mix garlic, rosemary, and oil in a small dish. Brush cutlets with mixture. Cook on a hot grill or barbecue. Boil sweet potato for 20 minutes, or until tender. Drain. Add remaining ingredients and mash until creamy. Combine salad vegetables and drizzle with vinegar, then toss through. Place sweet potato on plate and top with 3 cutlets per serve. Serve with corn salad.

Plan C variation
6 x 60g (360g) lamb cutlets, trimmed of fat

Nutritional analysis per serve	PLAN B	PLAN C
Energy (kJ)	2300	3054
Protein (g)	34	58
Fat (g)	25	34
Carbohydrate (g)	48	47
Fibre (g)	11	11
Sodium (mg)	336	418

Creamy Chicken Curry

Serves 2

1 medium potato, diced
15 green beans
⅓ cup tinned red lentils
½ small onion
250g skinless chicken breast, diced
1 tbsp curry powder
3 tsp cornflour
½ cup lite coconut cream
½ cup skim milk
⅔ cup basmati rice

Salsa
1 cup tomatoes, finely chopped
1 medium onion, finely chopped
1 small chilli, chopped

Combine salsa ingredients and set aside. Boil potato until tender. Steam beans. Rinse lentils in water.

In a large, non-stick frying pan, sauté onion, chicken, and curry powder until chicken is browned and cooked. Add vegetables. Heat for 3-4 minutes. Combine cornflour, coconut cream, and skim milk, then add to pan. Cook, stirring gently, over medium heat until thickened. Serve with cooked rice and salsa.

Plan C variation
500g skinless chicken breast

Nutritional analysis per serve	PLAN B	PLAN C
Energy (kJ)	2178	2963
Protein (g)	45	75
Fat (g)	14	22
Carbohydrate (g)	54	52
Fibre (g)	11	10
Sodium (mg)	211	302

Fish in Foil

Serves 2

300g Atlantic salmon, snapper, or barramundi fillet
1 tbsp olive oil
1 tbsp lemon juice
1 tbsp parsley, finely chopped
1 tbsp chives, finely chopped
1 clove garlic, crushed
8 cups garden salad

Place fish on a piece of foil. Brush or spray with oil and sprinkle with lemon juice, parsley, chives, and garlic. Wrap and bake at 180°C for 12-15 minutes, or until just pink in the centre. The fish will continue to cook once out of the oven. Serve with lemon slices and fresh garden salad.

Plan C variation
400g Atlantic salmon, snapper, or barramundi fillet

Nutritional analysis per serve	PLAN B	PLAN C
Energy (kJ)	1700	1997
Protein (g)	34	44
Fat (g)	21	25
Carbohydrate (g)	19	19
Fibre (g)	5	5
Sodium (mg)	98	120

Pork Stir-Fry

Serves 2

3 tsp canola oil
250g pork fillet, sliced
1 tsp sesame oil
4 cups fresh or frozen mixed stir-fry vegetables
2 tbsp soy sauce, salt-reduced
1 tbsp plum sauce

Heat half the oil on medium heat in a wok or frying pan. Stir-fry pork until browned. Remove, and set aside. Add remaining oils to pan. Stir-fry vegetables for about 4 minutes. Return pork to pan, add sauces and fry for 2 minutes, stirring. Serve and garnish with your choice of coriander, ginger, Thai basil, chilli, cashews, almonds, peanuts, sesame seeds, or pumpkin seeds.

Plan C variation
340g pork fillet, sliced

Nutritional analysis per serve	PLAN B	PLAN C
Energy (kJ)	1959	2254
Protein (g)	50	64
Fat (g)	14	16
Carbohydrate (g)	34	34
Fibre (g)	11	11
Sodium (mg)	996	1029

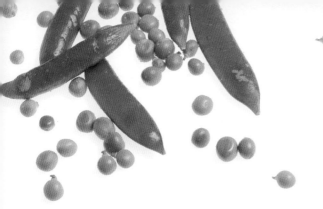

Chicken & Veg Soup

Serves 2

1L pre-prepared chicken stock, salt-reduced
250g chicken breast
1 tbsp canola oil
2 spring onions, finely chopped
3 cups fresh or frozen mixed vegetables
200g creamed corn
1 egg

Place stock in medium saucepan and bring
to boil. Slice chicken into small pieces and
add to stock. Reduce heat and simmer for
5 minutes. Add oil, spring onion (save a little
for garnish), vegetables, and corn. Heat
through. Beat egg. Just before serving soup,
add egg and stir. Garnish with spring onions.

Plan C variation
300g chicken breast

Note: *This recipe can be doubled to serve 4
and frozen for convenience.*

Nutritional analysis per serve	PLAN B	PLAN C
Energy (kJ)	1720	2234
Protein (g)	40	48
Fat (g)	11	13
Carbohydrate (g)	37	55
Fibre (g)	12	16
Sodium (mg)	1380	1736

Steak & Vegetables

Serves 2

340g rump, scotch, fillet or T-bone steak,
  trimmed of fat
1 tbsp olive oil
1 cup pumpkin
1½ cups peas
1 cup yellow baby squash or cauliflower
1 cup broccoli

Brush steak with oil and place on grill.
A medium-rare steak that is 2.5cm thick
should be grilled for 4-5 minutes on both
sides. Place vegetables in microwave-proof
bowl and cook on high for 5 minutes, or
until cooked through. For a flavour boost,
marinate steak in your favourite herbs and
spices, e.g., Moroccan spice mix, Cajun spice
mix, or chilli and lemon pepper.

Plan C variation
480g rump, scotch, fillet or T-bone steak,
trimmed of fat

Nutritional analysis per serve	PLAN B	PLAN C
Energy (kJ)	1765	2142
Protein (g)	48	64
Fat (g)	18	21
Carbohydrate (g)	17	17
Fibre (g)	10	10
Sodium (mg)	93	125

Tuna & Veg Frittata

Serves 2

1 tbsp olive oil
½ red onion
½ medium zucchini, grated or thinly sliced
90g tinned tuna
2 cups mixed frozen vegetables
1 tbsp mixed herbs
3 tomatoes, chopped roughly
4 eggs
⅓ cup low-fat ricotta cheese
¼ tsp black pepper
4 cups mixed salad greens

Preheat grill. Heat oil in non-stick frying pan and cook onion and zucchini until soft. Add tuna, mixed vegetables, herbs, and half the tomatoes. Cook for another 2-3 minutes. Beat egg and cheese together and pour over mixture. Cook on medium heat for 4-5 minutes until base is brown and top nearly set. Sprinkle with pepper and place under grill until golden. To make salad, combine salad greens with remaining tomatoes. Slice frittata and serve hot with side salad.

Plan C variation
6 eggs

Nutritional analysis per serve	PLAN B	PLAN C
Energy (kJ)	1802	2157
Protein (g)	30	43
Fat (g)	21	25
Carbohydrate (g)	29	29
Fibre (g)	8	8
Sodium (mg)	231	297

Chinese Steamed Fish

Serves 2

1 tbsp sesame oil
2 tbsp soy sauce
½ tsp garlic, crushed
1 tsp ginger, grated
1 tsp sugar
500g ocean perch
2 cup snowpeas
1 cup broccoli florets
2 cups bok choy, chopped
1 medium shallot, sliced
½ tsp sesame seeds

Combine sesame oil, soy sauce, garlic, ginger, and sugar to make dressing. Place fish on a plate and pour over half the dressing. Cover with plastic film. Steam in microwave for about 8 minutes on high, longer if fillets are thick. Steam snowpeas, broccoli, and bok choy in a microwave-proof container on high for 3-4 minutes.

To serve: Arrange fish and vegetables on plates. Pour over remaining dressing and sprinkle with sliced shallots and sesame seeds.

Plan C variation
750g ocean perch

Nutritional analysis per serve	PLAN B	PLAN C
Energy (kJ)	1388	1773
Protein (g)	49	70
Fat (g)	12	12
Carbohydrate (g)	7	7
Fibre (g)	5	5
Sodium (mg)	918	999

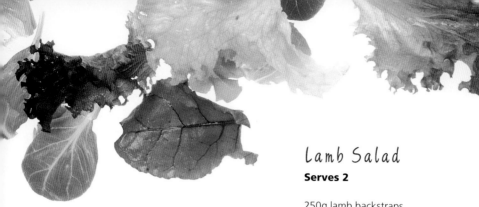

Beef & Black Bean BBQ

Serves 2

250g beef steak, trimmed of fat, thinly sliced
1 medium brown onion, finely diced
2 cups bok choy, chopped
2 celery stalks, thinly sliced
1 cup snowpeas
1 tbsp peanut oil (or sesame or canola)
1 clove garlic, crushed
¼ cup black bean sauce, salt-reduced
1 tbsp plum sauce

Heat oil on barbecue plate and brown beef on all sides. Remove and set aside. Barbecue onion, garlic, and celery until softened. Add bok choy, snowpeas, and sauces. Cook until sauce boils. Return beef to plate, mix with vegetables, and serve immediately.

Plan C variation
340g beef steak, trimmed of fat and thinly sliced

Nutritional analysis per serve	PLAN B	PLAN C
Energy (kJ)	1719	2033
Protein (g)	40	53
Fat (g)	20	22
Carbohydrate (g)	19	19
Fibre (g)	5	5
Sodium (mg)	475	502

Lamb Salad

Serves 2

250g lamb backstraps
olive oil spray
4 green onions, thinly sliced
2 cups fresh flat-leaf parsley, chopped
1 cup tomatoes, chopped
½ cup kalamata olives, pitted
4 cups green salad leaves, torn

Dressing
2 tsp olive oil
1 clove garlic, crushed
juice of 1 lemon
pinch of salt and pepper

Preheat pan and spray with olive oil. Cook lamb, turning occasionally, until cooked. Set aside to rest for 10 minutes. Combine onions, parsley, tomatoes, and olives in a large bowl. In a jar with a tight lid, combine oil, garlic, lemon juice, salt and pepper, and shake. Slice lamb and add to tomato mixture. Pour over dressing. Toss to combine and serve on a bed of salad leaves.

Plan C variation
340g lamb backstraps

Nutritional analysis per serve	PLAN B	PLAN C
Energy (kJ)	1605	1942
Protein (g)	42	55
Fat (g)	18	21
Carbohydrate (g)	13	13
Fibre (g)	6	6
Sodium (mg)	400	437

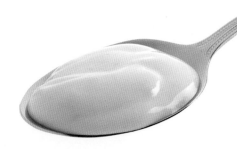

Chicken & Ginger

Serves 2

300g chicken breast
1½ tbsp fresh ginger, grated
1 tbsp olive oil
1 tomato, diced
¼ red capsicum, diced
4 cups fresh or frozen mixed green vegetables

Place chicken on foil. Combine 1 tablespoon ginger with half the oil and spread over top of chicken. Fold foil to seal and place in a preheated moderate oven. After 25 minutes, remove from oven and slice open foil. Return it to oven and brown for 10 minutes. Combine tomato, capsicum, remaining ginger, and olive oil in microwave-proof bowl. Cover and cook for 45 seconds on high. Use a bamboo steamer or microwave to steam green vegetables. Serve chicken topped with salsa with a side of steamed vegetables.

Plan C variation
400g chicken breast

Nutritional analysis per serve	PLAN B	PLAN C
Energy (kJ)	1989	2305
Protein (g)	46	57
Fat (g)	20	23
Carbohydrate (g)	28	28
Fibre (g)	12	12
Sodium (mg)	147	178

Vegetable Omelette

Serves 2

6 eggs
1 tbsp skim milk
2 tsp plain flour
130g can creamed corn
3 cups frozen mixed vegetables,
    thawed and drained
¼ tsp ground nutmeg
250g packet of frozen spinach, thawed
1 tbsp olive oil

Whisk eggs, milk, and flour together in a bowl. Stir in corn, vegetables, and nutmeg. Squeeze excess moisture from spinach and stir into egg mixture. Heat oil in a non-stick frying pan. Pour half the mixture into pan. Cook until omelette is almost set, then fold in half. Cook for a further minute, remove and keep warm. Repeat with remaining mixture.

Plan C variation
8 eggs

Nutritional analysis per serve	PLAN B	PLAN C
Energy (kJ)	2099	2396
Protein (g)	33	40
Fat (g)	26	31
Carbohydrate (g)	34	34
Fibre (g)	17	17
Sodium (mg)	567	634

Tandoori Chicken

Serves 2

300g chicken tenderloins
100g low-fat natural yoghurt
1 tsp minced garlic
2 tsp tandoori mix
1 tomato, finely chopped
½ Lebanese cucumber, finely chopped
1 small red onion
1 tbsp lemon juice
6 cups mixed salad greens

Cut each tenderloin into pieces, and thread onto skewers. Preheat foil-lined grill or barbecue grill plate to moderately hot. Combine yoghurt, garlic, and tandoori mix, then spoon or brush over chicken. Cook skewers for 10 minutes, turning once after 5 minutes. Combine tomato, cucumber, onion, lemon juice, and salad greens. Serve the skewers with garden salad and yoghurt.

Plan C variation
400g chicken tenderloins

Nutritional analysis per serve	PLAN B	PLAN C
Energy (kJ)	1926	2378
Protein (g)	46	59
Fat (g)	21	27
Carbohydrate (g)	21	21
Fibre (g)	6	6
Sodium (mg)	229	282

SNACKS AND EXTRAS
Plans B and C

Sweet Snacks

150g tub low-fat fruit yoghurt
1 low-fat banana smoothie
1 plain muesli bar (no yoghurt or chocolate topping)
1 breakfast bar
1 fruit scone with 1 teaspoon jam
200ml low-fat flavoured milk
2 small pikelets with 2 teaspoons jam
1 slice mixed grain fruit loaf with 1 teaspoon jam
1 cup fruit salad with 2 tablespoons low-fat fruit yoghurt
1 cup fruit salad with 1 scoop low-fat ice-cream
30g dried fruit and nut mix
2 medium apples
1 mango
2 small bananas
1 slice of apple strudel
150g serve of low-fat creamed rice pudding
1 banana and oat bran muffin

Savoury Snacks

2 rice cakes with 2 teaspoons light cream cheese
12 rice crackers with salsa dip
10 hot chips
35g pretzels
2 tablespoons peanuts
3 cups air-popped popcorn with 1 teaspoon margarine
1 slice multigrain toast with 2 tablespoons baked beans

Extras

no more than 3 a week

small packet potato chips (25g)
1 plain chocolate ice-cream on a stick
1½ chocolate biscuits
2 fingers of a wafer chocolate bar
1 small piece of boiled fruit cake
200ml wine
375ml beer

contract of commitment

This contract is entered into on _____ **by and between Fitsmart**
(date)
and _____.
(name)

1. Terms and Condition

By agreeing to sign up to a Fitsmart Weight Loss program,
I hereby commit to the following long-term goals:

1.1_____

1.2_____

1.3_____

2. Time Period

I agree to nominate a set time period in which to fulfil all the terms of this contract,
which is as follows:

2.1_____

3. Benefits

In agreeing to the terms of this contract, and fulfilling my duties, I intend to receive the
following benefits:

3.1_____

3.2_____

3.3_____

4. Acceptance of Term and Conditions

I,_____, understand and accept the terms
and conditions outlined above.

_____   _____
(Signature and date)   **(Name)**

_____   Guy Leech_____

FOOD AND FITNESS RESULTS

Use this chart to record your answers and results from the Getting Started chapter. Record everything as it is now, as it's a great way to keep yourself motivated if you've got a starting point to refer back to. Be sure to retest yourself in a month's time—there's no doubt you'll surprise yourself with how far you've come. And congratulate yourself for every change that takes place, no matter how small—it's still a success and it's something to be proud of.

Measurements		Now		Wk 4		Wk 8	
		Now		Wk 4		Wk 8	
		Now		Wk 4		Wk 8	
		Now		Wk 4		Wk 8	
Fitness		Now		Wk 4		Wk 8	
		Now		Wk 4		Wk 8	
		Now		Wk 4		Wk 8	
		Now		Wk 4		Wk 8	

	Body Fat Percentage		Hips		Mid Bicep		Mid Thigh		Chest	
RESULTS OF:	Step Up	2.4km Run		Abdominal Strength	Upper Torso Strength			Sit and Reach		

FOOD AND FITNESS DIARY

Use these pages to record your progress while you're on your tailored Fitsmart System 3 program. You should have your overall goal in mind, but make sure you fill in your weekly goals to make it even easier to reach. Make a time each week to sit down by yourself and fill in your diary, recording all the exercise for that week, the meals and quantities you intend to eat, and anything that needs to be focused on, and then tick them off as you go.

Before filling in these pages, you may want to make copies of them so you'll have enough for your entire program, and beyond. Alternatively, you can visit our website **www.fitsmart.com.au** and follow the links to the printable copies of these diary pages.

THIS WEEK'S GOALS	2 laps of oval							✓
	10 laps of the pool							
	Eat more fruit							
	Start jogging in the morning							

	MON	TUE	WED	THURS	FRI	SAT	SUN
EXERCISE PLAN	push-ups 12 ✓						
Breakfast	muesli ✓						
Morning snack	Apple Bar ✓						
Lunch	salad ✓						
Afternoon snack	fruit ✗						
Dinner	Penne ✓						
Supper							
DRINKS AND WATER CONSUMED THIS WEEK	water x3						
	wine x3						
EXTRA FOOD EATEN THIS WEEK	pie, donut						
	burger n fries						
3 AREAS OF HEALTHY EATING QUESTIONNAIRE TO BE WORKED ON							

THIS WEEK'S GOALS							
	MON	**TUE**	**WED**	**THURS**	**FRI**	**SAT**	**SUN**
EXERCISE PLAN							
Breakfast							
Morning snack							
Lunch							
Afternoon snack							
Dinner							
Supper							
DRINKS AND WATER CONSUMED THIS WEEK							
EXTRA FOOD EATEN THIS WEEK							
3 AREAS OF HEALTHY EATING QUESTIONNAIRE TO BE WORKED ON